LANGE

USMLE
ROAD MAP
IMMUNOLOGY

Notice

LANGE

USMLE ROAD MAP

IMMUNOLOGY

MICHAEL J. PARMELY, PhD

Professor
Department of Microbiology, Molecular Genetics and Immunology
University of Kansas Medical Center
Kansas City, Kansas

Lange Medical Books/McGraw-Hill
Medical Publishing Division

New York   Chicago   San Francisco   Lisbon   London   Madrid   Mexico City
Milan   New Delhi   San Juan   Seoul   Singapore   Sydney   Toronto

The **McGraw·Hill** Companies

USMLE Road Map: Immunology

1234567890 DOC/DOC 09876

ISBN: 0-07-145298-2

ISSN: 1559-5765

This book was set in Adobe Garamond by Pine Tree Composition, Inc.
The editors were Jason Malley, Harriet Lebowitz, and Mary E. Bele.
The production supervisor was Sherri Souffrance.
The illustration manager was Charissa Baker.
The illustrator was Dragonfly Media Group.
The designer was Eve Siegel.
The index was prepared by Andover Publishing Services.
RR Donnelley was printer and binder.

This book is printed on acid-free paper.

INTERNATIONAL EDITION ISBN 0-07-110477-1 Copyright © 2006. Exclusive right by The McGraw-Hill Companies, Inc. for manufacture and export. This book cannot be re-exported from the country to which it is consigned by McGraw-Hill. The International Edition is not available in North America.

CONTENTS

USING THE
USMLE ROAD MAP SERIES
FOR SUCCESSFUL REVIEW

What Is the Road Map Series?

Short of having your own personal tutor, the USMLE Road Map Series is the best source for efficient review of major concepts and information in the medical sciences.

Why Do You Need A Road Map?

It allows you to navigate quickly and easily through your immunology course notes and textbook and prepares you for USMLE and course examinations.

How Does the Road Map Series Work?

Outline Form: Connects the facts in a conceptual framework so that you understand the ideas and retain the information.

Color and Boldface: Highlights words and phrases that trigger quick retrieval of concepts and facts.

Clear Explanations: Are fine-tuned by years of student interaction. The material is written by authors selected for their excellence in teaching and their experience in preparing students for board examinations.

Illustrations: Provide the vivid impressions that facilitate comprehension and recall.

 Clinical Correlations: Link all topics to their clinical applications, promoting fuller understanding and memory retention.

 Clinical Problems: Give you valuable practice for the clinical vignette-based USMLE questions.

 Explanations of Answers: Are learning tools that allow you to pinpoint your strengths and weaknesses.

Acknowledgments

Special thanks go to my colleagues, Thomas Yankee, Kevin Latinis, Glenn Mackay, and David Cue, for their careful review of selected chapters. I am grateful to Harriet Lebowitz for her editorial advice and assistance.

To Tari, for her constant love, patience, and support.
To my students, who teach me something new every day.

CHAPTER 1
INNATE IMMUNITY

I. Immunity is distinguished by the following features.

A. The immune system, which protects the body against microbial invaders and environmental agents, takes two forms.

  1. Innate immunity is available at birth and protects the newborn from pathogenic microbes.

  2. Adaptive or acquired immunity arises in the host as a consequence of exposure to a microbe or foreign substance.

B. The life-style of the microbe determines the nature of the protective immune response.

  1. Extracellular microbes can be neutralized by antibodies and other soluble immune mediators.

  2. Elimination of **intracellular pathogens** requires their recognition by immune cells that can destroy pathogen-infected host cells.

C. Both forms of immunity require a specific recognition of the pathogen or environmental agent and an ability to distinguish it from "self."

D. Innate immunity is a phylogenetically ancient defense mechanism designed for rapidly recognizing, lysing, or phagocytozing pathogenic microbes and signaling their presence to the host.

  1. The innate immune system recognizes **microbial patterns** that are widely distributed across genera, rather than the discrete antigenic determinants that characterize a particular species of microbe (Chapter 2).

  2. Innate immunity does not require prior exposure to the offending agent and is not altered by a previous encounter with it.

  3. Innate immunity is expressed within minutes to hours, representing the first response of the host to microbial pathogens.

E. The **effector mechanisms** used by the innate immune system to eliminate foreign invaders (eg, phagocytosis) are often the same as those used for immune elimination during an adaptive immune response (Chapter 2).

F. Many of the responses we consider to be part of the innate immune system also play a central role in **inflammatory responses** to tissue injury (Table 1–1).

II. First lines of defense limit microbial survival.

A. Physical and chemical barriers provide some of the first lines of innate defense by preventing microbial attachment, entry, or local tissue survival in a nonspecific manner.

1

Table 1–1. Components shared by the innate immune and inflammatory systems.

Component	Innate Immune Effects	Inflammatory Effects
Phagocytic leukocytes	Intracellular killing of microbes	Elimination of damaged host cells
Complement system	Chemoattraction of leukocytes Lysis, opsonophagocytosis and clearance of microbes	Chemoattraction of leukocytes Increased vascular permeability
Fibrinolysis system	Complement activation Leukocyte chemotaxis	Increased vascular permeability Leukocyte chemotaxis
Vascular endothelium	Delivery of immune mediators to sites of infection	Delivery of inflammatory mediators to sites of damaged tissues
Cytokines	Danger signaling Phagocyte activation Respiratory burst Fever	Leukocyte adhesion, chemotaxis, and uptake of cellular debris Phagocyte activation Fever Tissue healing
Neutrophil granules	Antimicrobial cationic peptides	Extracellular matrix degradation

1. The **epithelium** of the skin and mucous membranes provides a physical barrier.
2. The **mucocilliary movement** of the lung epithelium and the **peristalsis** of the gastrointestinal tract move microbes and other foreign agents across mucosal surfaces and out of the body.
3. The **low pH** and high fatty acid content of the skin inhibit microbial growth.
4. The low pH of the stomach damages essential structures of microbes and limits their survival.
5. **Mucins** associated with mucosal epithelia prevent microbial penetration and bind soluble immune factors (eg, antibody molecules).
6. A variety of **iron-binding proteins** (eg, lactoferrin) compete with microbes for extracellular iron.
   a. Lactoferrin competes for iron in the extracellular space.
   b. The *Nramp1* gene product enables host cells to acquire the Fe^{2+} ions necessary to generate reactive oxygen species.
   c. *Nramp2* aids cells in depleting Fe^{2+} from the phagosome, thus inhibiting microbial survival.

B. The **normal flora** found at epithelial surfaces provides a **biological barrier** to pathogenic microbes that attempt to survive at that site.
   1. Normal microbial flora competes with pathogens for nutrients and environmental niches, especially at external body surfaces, such as the skin, intestines, and lungs.
   2. Normal flora can induce innate immune responses in the epithelium that limit the survival of pathogenic microorganisms.

III. Pathogens that breach the primary barriers initiate an innate immune response.

A. **Pathogen-associated molecular patterns** (PAMP) are recognized by innate immune cells and soluble mediators.

1. PAMP are often highly charged surface structures or unique spatial arrangements of chemical groups (eg, sugar moieties) that are not seen on host tissues.

2. PAMP are phylogenetically conserved structures that are essential for the survival of microorganisms.

3. Host cell receptors capable of recognizing PAMP are encoded within the germline and are phylogenetically conserved.

a. Relatively few host cell surface receptors are required to recognize a wide range of pathogens.

b. The **Toll-like receptor** (TLR) family is an important example of phylogenetically conserved PAMP-specific host molecules (Table 1–2).

4. A number of soluble host proteins also recognize PAMP.

a. **Mannose-binding protein** (MBP) (also called **mannose-binding lectin**) binds to mannose residues of a particular spacing that is seen on microbial, but not mammalian, cells.

(1) MBP serves as an opsonin promoting phagocytosis.

(2) MBP promotes lysis and phagocytosis of microbes by activating complement (Chapter 8).

b. **Lysozyme** degrades the peptidoglycan layer of bacterial cell walls.

Table 1–2. The Toll-like receptor (TLR) family.

TLR	Microbial Ligands
TLR1	Bacterial lipopeptides
TLR2	Bacterial peptidoglycan, lipoteichoic acid, lipoarabinomannan, glycolipids, porins
TLR3	Viral double-stranded RNA
TLR4	Bacterial lipopolysaccharide, viral proteins
TLR5	Bacterial flagellin
TLR6	Bacterial lipopeptides; fungal cell wall
TLR7	Viral single-stranded RNA
TLR8	Viral single-stranded RNA
TLR9	Bacterial CpG-containing DNA

B. The recognition of PAMP activates leukocyte functions.

1. Phagocytic **leukocytes** (blood neutrophils and tissue macrophages) can recognize microbes directly through their **mannose receptors, scavenger receptors, Toll-like receptors**, or **chemotactic receptors**.

   a. The recognition of microbial **chemotactic factors** directs leukocytes to the site of infection.

      (1) Chemotactic factors can be either microbial or host in origin (Table 1–3).

      (2) Chemotactic factors are recognized by seven transmembrane G protein-coupled **receptors**.

   b. Opsonic receptors on leukocytes recognize host components that have bound to the surface of microbes.

   c. Attachment of a microbe to the surface of a phagocyte is followed by its **uptake** by membrane invagination (Figure 1–1).

      (1) The microbe is ingested into a **phagosome**.

      (2) The **phagosome** fuses with an organelle called the **lysosome** to form a **phagolysosome**.

   d. Intracellular killing of the microbe occurs within the phagolysosome.

      (1) Lysosomal **hydrolytic enzymes** (acidic proteases, lipases, and nucleases) degrade microbial structures.

      (2) Leukocyte cytoplasmic granules containing cationic antimicrobial peptides (**defensins** and **cathelicidins**) fuse with the phagolysosome.

         (a) These peptides act as disinfectants by disrupting the membrane functions of microorganisms.

         (b) Defensins recognize the highly charged phospholipids on the outer membranes of microbes.

         (c) Antimicrobial peptides of very similar structure have been found both in the vernix caseosa covering the skin of newborn humans and the skin secretions of frogs.

Table 1–3. Chemotactic factors that attract innate immune cells.

Cell Type	Chemotactic Factors
Neutrophil	Bacterial lipoteichoic acid Bacterial formyl-methionyl peptides Complement peptide C5a Fibrinogen-derived peptides Leukotriene B$_4$ Mast cell-derived chemotactic peptide NCF-A Cytokines: interleukin-8
Macrophage	Cytokines: transforming growth factor-β, monocyte chemotactic protein-1
Lymphocyte	Cytokines: macrophage inflammatory protein-1

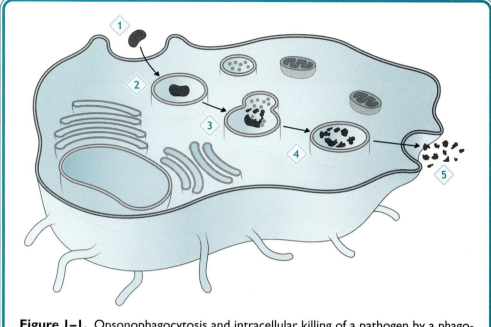

Figure 1–1. Opsonophagocytosis and intracellular killing of a pathogen by a phagocytic cell. 1, Attachment; 2, ingestion (phagosome); 3, phagolysosome; 4, killing, digestion; 5, release.

(3) In the presence of adequate oxygen, microbe recognition at the phagocytic cell surface can initiate a **respiratory burst**, the one electron reduction of molecular oxygen (Figure 1–2).

(a) **Reactive oxygen intermediates** (oxidants and radicals) produced during this process irreversibly damage essential microbial structures.

(b) The reaction begins with the **respiratory burst oxidase**, a multicomponent membrane-associated enzyme.

(c) This oxidase catalyzes the reduction of oxygen (O_2) to the radical **superoxide** ($O_2^{\bullet}$).

(d) The dismutation of superoxide to form **hydrogen peroxide** (H_2O_2) is catalyzed by the enzyme **superoxide dismutase** (SOD).

(e) In the presence of a halide (eg, chloride ion), neutrophil-specific **myeloperoxidase** catalyzes the production of hypohalite (eg, **hypochlorite** or bleach) and organic chloramines.

(f) In the presence of ferric ion, the highly reactive **hydroxyl radical** ($OH^{\bullet}$) is formed from superoxide and hydrogen peroxide.

CHRONIC GRANULOMATOUS DISEASE (CGD) IS A MUTATION OF THE RESPIRATORY BURST OXIDASE

• Mutations in the subunits of the **respiratory burst oxidase** (also called NADPH oxidase) can lead to a decreased production of the superoxide radical by phagocytes.

CLINICAL CORRELATION

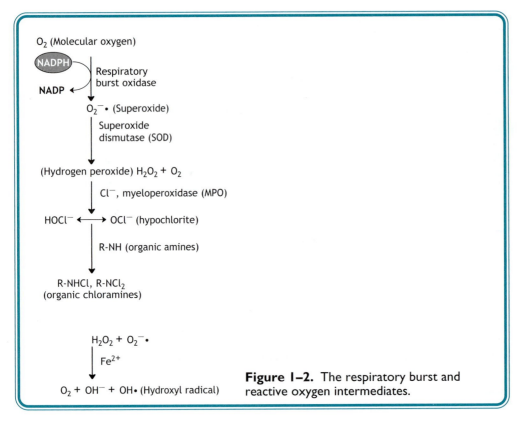

O_2 (Molecular oxygen)

NADPH

NADP

Respiratory burst oxidase

$O_2^-\bullet$ (Superoxide)

Superoxide dismutase (SOD)

(Hydrogen peroxide) $H_2O_2 + O_2$

Cl^-, myeloperoxidase (MPO)

$HOCl^- \longleftrightarrow OCl^-$ (hypochlorite)

R-NH (organic amines)

R-NHCl, R-NCl$_2$
(organic chloramines)

$H_2O_2 + O_2^-\bullet$

Fe^{2+}

$O_2 + OH^- + OH\bullet$ (Hydroxyl radical)

Figure 1–2. The respiratory burst and reactive oxygen intermediates.

- *Leukocytes of CGD patients fail to produce many of the oxidants that mediate killing of microorganisms within the phagolysosome.*
- *CGD patients are at risk for acquiring **opportunistic infections** with microbes that would otherwise show low virulence in normal individuals.*
- *Because the phagocytosis of microbes is normal in these patients, some pathogens that are not killed replicate within the phagolysosome.*
- *The host attempts to wall off leukocytes containing viable microbes by forming a structure called a **granuloma** in the lungs and liver.*

   (4) Oxygen-independent intracellular killing is essential when tissue oxygen is limited, as in deep tissue abscesses.

   (5) Some phagocytic cells (eg, tissue macrophages) produce the radical **nitric oxide (NO•)**, which can damage microbial structures.

    (a) NO• is formed from L-arginine and oxygen through a reaction catalyzed by **nitric oxide synthase (NOS)**:

L-arginine-NH$_2$ + NADPH + O$_2$ → NO• + L-citruline + NADP

    (b) In macrophages and hepatocytes, the **inducible form of NOS (iNOS)** catalyzes high level, sustained production of NO• that functions as an antimicrobial agent.

    (c) Only a few microbes (eg, *Mycobacteria* and *Listeria* species) are highly susceptible to NO•.

(*d*) When $NO^\bullet$ and $O_2^\bullet$ combine, they form **peroxynitrite** ($ONOO^-$), an especially potent oxidant.

2. **Epithelial cells also produce the defensins.**
   a. Defensins limit microbial survival at the mucosal surface of the lung, intestine, and genitourinary tract.
   b. Defensins are chemotactic for dendritic cells, monocytes, and T lymphocytes that mediate mucosal defense.
3. **Intraepithelial T lymphocytes** are found in the skin, lung, and small intestine.
   a. These cells bear germline gene-encoded antigen receptors (Chapter 6) that recognize conserved microbial glycolipids.
   b. Intraepithelial T cells mediate host protection by the secretion of cytokines that can activate phagocytic cells.
4. **Natural killer (NK) cells** recognize host cells that are infected with intracellular pathogens, such as viruses.
   a. NK cells bear two types of receptors, one for activating the cell and another for inhibiting its activation.
      (*1*) NK cell **activating receptors** are specific for host and microbial ligands.
      (*2*) NK cell **inhibitory receptors** are specific for **major histocompatibility complex (MHC)** molecules that are widely distributed on host tissues (Chapter 7).
      (*3*) When the inhibitory receptor binds host MHC molecules, activation of the NK cell is blocked.
      (*4*) When the expression of MHC molecules is decreased on host tissues, NK cells become activated through their activating receptors.
      (*5*) The expression of MHC is often decreased on virus-infected cells.
   b. Upon activation, NK cells can eliminate microbial pathogens by secreting cytokines, which activate macrophages.
   c. NK cells can also lyse infected host cells.
   d. NK cells also synthesize **interferons** (Chapter 12) that block the replication of viruses within infected cells.
5. **Natural killer T (NKT) cells** bear many of the surface receptors present on NK cells as well as an unconventional form of the **T cell antigen receptor** (Chapter 6).
   a. Most NKT cells are specific for microbial glycolipids.
   b. NKT cells can produce cytokines capable of activating macrophages.
   c. NKT cells can express cytotoxic activity, although the role of this function in host defense is still unclear.
C. The recognition of microbial pathogens signals "danger" to the host.
   1. **TLRs** (Table 1–2) initiate danger signaling when they bind microbial PAMP.
      a. Intracellular signal transduction initiated by TLR leads to the activation of transcription factors.
      b. For example, **TLR4** mediates the recognition of bacterial **lipopolysaccharides (LPS)**, which are common components of the outer membrane of gram-negative bacteria (Figure 1–3)
      c. TLR4 signaling results in the activation of the **nuclear factor-κB (NFκB)** and **AP-1** transcription factors.
      d. Among the genes regulated by NFκB and AP-1 are those encoding proinflammatory cytokines and their receptors, cell adhesion molecules, immunoglobulins, and antigen receptors.

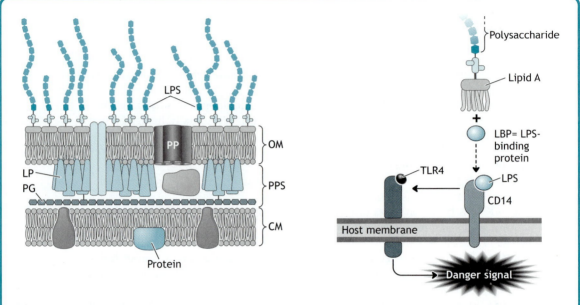

Figure 1–3. Cellular responses to bacterial lipopolysaccharide (LPS) are mediated by toll-like receptor 4 (TLR4). CM, cytoplasmic membrane; LP, lipoprotein; LPS, lipopolysaccharide; OM, outer membrane; PG, peptidoglycan; PP, porin protein; PPS, periplasmic space.

EXCESSIVE DANGER SIGNALING AND SEPSIS

- *Sepsis is a systemic host response to disseminated infection characterized by fever, tachycardia, tachypnea, hemodynamic dysfunction, coagulopathy, and multiorgan damage.*
- *These processes result from microvascular changes, diminished tissue perfusion, and inadequate tissue oxygenation.*
- *Sepsis represents excessive danger signaling on the part of the host; soluble and cellular mediators of innate immunity are produced in excess.*
- *The cytokines interleukin (IL)-1, interferon (IFN)-γ, and tumor necrosis factor (TNF)-α are important early mediators of sepsis.*
- *Clinical trials using reagents (eg, antibodies) designed to neutralize any one of these mediators have been disappointing, probably owing to mediator redundancy.*

    2. Cytokine genes are induced by danger signaling and are essential for appropriate innate immune responses to infection.

       a. Cytokines are peptide hormone-like mediators of immunity and inflammation (Chapter 12).

       b. Cytokines are produced by a variety of immune cells and induce gene expression, cell growth, and differentiation.

       c. Cytokines act through specific **cytokine receptors**, many of which activate gene transcription.

       d. Among the important effects of cytokines are fever, hematopoiesis, chemotaxis, increased cell adhesion, changes in blood vessel function, antibody production, and apoptosis (Table 1–4).

Table 1–4. Cytokines that act as danger signals.[a]

Cytokine	Functions Related to Danger Signaling
TNF-α	Fever, leukocyte adhesion to endothelium, acute phase protein synthesis, respiratory burst, cachexia, cardiac suppression, disseminated intravascular coagulation and shock
IL-1, IL-6	Fever, leukocyte adhesion to endothelium, acute phase protein synthesis, B lymphocyte coactivation
Chemokines	Lymphocyte and leukocyte migration to sites of infection
IL-4	Lymphocyte coactivation and antibody production
IL-12	Lymphocyte coactivation and cell-mediated immunity
IFN-α, IFN-β	Antiviral state, coactivation of macrophages and NK cells, increased MHC expression
IFN-γ	Coactivation of macrophages, increased MHC expression

[a]TNF, tumor necrosis factor; IL, interleukin; IFN, interferon; NK, natural killer; MHC, major histocompatibility complex.

  e. The **interferons (IFN)** are a family of cytokines first noted for their antiviral activity.
   (1) IFN-α and IFN-β block virus replication within cells.
   (2) IFN-γ is a potent activator of macrophages for the killing of intracellular bacteria and fungi.

DEFECTIVE IFN-γ RECEPTOR FUNCTION LEADS TO OPPORTUNISTIC INFECTIONS

CLINICAL CORRELATION

- *The killing of intracellular microbial pathogens by macrophages requires that the cells be activated by microbial or host signals, including cytokines.*
- *IFN-γ is a potent macrophage activating cytokine that acts on cells through its receptor.*
- *Point mutations in the human IFN-γ receptor 1 gene impair signaling and macrophage activation for the killing of intracellular pathogens.*
- *Life-threatening infections with Mycobacterium and Salmonella species are common and can become widely disseminated throughout the body.*
- *Because the receptors for IFN-α and IFN-β are distinct from those that bind IFN-γ, the affected individuals do not suffer from increased viral infections.*

  3. PAMP can activate the **complement** system of serum proteins.
   a. Several complement components can recognize highly charged microbial structures, such as bacterial LPS and surface mannose residues.

b. Peptides produced during complement activation mediate host defense and inflammatory functions, such as the chemotaxis of neutrophils, opsonization, and the lysis of microbial membranes.

   c. The activation of mast cell degranulation by complement peptides, called **anaphylatoxins**, leads to the release of an additional wave of inflammatory mediators that are stored in mast cell cytoplasmic granules (Chapter 13).

4. The synthesis of **acute phase proteins** is a response to danger signaling.

   a. Many acute phase proteins are produced in the liver in response to the cytokines IL-1, IL-6, and TNF-α.

   b. **C-reactive protein (CRP)** binds to bacterial surface phospholipids, activates complement, and serves as an opsonin.

   c. Increased **fibrinogen** in plasma increases the **erythrocyte sedimentation rate (ESR)**, a clinical laboratory test indicative of acute inflammation.

5. The **coagulation** and **fibrinolysis** systems are activated during acute infections and inflammation.

   a. Coagulation serves to localize infection by retaining microbes within a fibrin clot.

   b. Peptides derived from fibrinogen during fibrinolysis are chemotactic for neutrophils.

   c. **Plasmin** generated during fibrinolysis can activate the complement system.

DYSREGULATION OF THE COMPLEMENT SYSTEM RESULTS IN ACUTE INFLAMMATION

- *Unabated activation of the complement system is potentially harmful to the host due to the production of inflammatory mediators.*
- *An important regulator of the classic pathway of complement activation is the protease inhibitor **C1 inhibitor (C1 !nh)**.*
- *Patients with **hereditary angioedema (HAE)** have significantly decreased levels of plasma C1 Inh.*
- *Episodic activation of complement in HAE patients results in the production of complement peptides that increase vascular permeability.*
- *The resulting subcutaneous and submucosal edema can lead to airway obstruction, asphyxiation, and severe abdominal pain.*

IV. Danger signals can promote the activation of antigen-specific T and B lymphocytes of the adaptive immune system.

   A. The nature of danger signaling depends on the type of microbe.

   1. Intracellular pathogens often induce innate signals (eg, IL-12) that promote the development of cellular immunity.

   2. Extracellular pathogens often favor induction of antibody responses to microbial antigens (Chapter 2).

   B. Danger signals activate T and B lymphocytes through their cell surface **coreceptors**.

   1. The complement peptide C3d generated during an innate immune response is the ligand for the **B cell coreceptor CR2**.

   2. C3d costimulates B cells that have bound antigen through their antigen receptors (Chapter 8).

C. Cytokines produced by innate immune cells are important regulators of lymphocyte activation during adaptive immune responses.
    1. IFN-α and IFN-β enhance T lymphocyte responses to microbial antigens by controlling the expression of MHC molecules (Chapter 7).
    2. IL-4 and IL-5 promote the production of certain classes of antibodies by B lymphocytes.
    3. IL-12 promotes differentiation of T lymphocytes.

D. Adjuvants are substances that promote adaptive immune responses.
    1. Most adjuvants act by inducing danger signaling.
    2. Adjuvants can increase the expression of lymphocyte coreceptors.
    3. Adjuvants can induce the expression of ligands for lymphocyte coreceptors.
    4. Adjuvants can induce cytokine production or increased cytokine receptor expression.

CLINICAL PROBLEMS

Ms. Jones is a retired secretary who has been admitted to the hospital for treatment of an apparent urinary tract infection. She is administered a third-generation cephalosporin antibiotic at approximately 1:00 PM, at which time she has a fever of 101°F, blood pressure of 110/60, and a pulse of 115. The patient tolerates the antibiotic well during the first hour, but when the nurse returns to her room at 3:00 PM, Ms. Jones' vital signs have deteriorated. Her blood pressure has decreased to 80/50, her pulse is now 128, and she no longer responds when called by name. Her physician concludes that Ms. Jones is septic.

1. Which of the following treatments should be administered immediately?

    A. Increase the dose of antibiotic to control the infection.

    B. Administer a vasodilator, such as verapamil.

    C. Discontinue the antibiotic and administer intravenous fluids.

    D. Administer TNF-α to control the infection.

    E. Administer complement components to control the systemic inflammatory response.

Johnny is a 1-month-old healthy child who has not, as yet, received any childhood immunizations. He presents with his first episode of otitis media (middle ear infection) that is successfully treated with a 3-week course of antibiotics.

2. Which one of the following immune components contributed the most to his clearing the infectious agent during the first few days of his infection?

    A. Antigen receptors on his B lymphocytes

    B. Toll-like receptors on his neutrophils

    C. Cytokines that promoted antibody formation

    D. T cell responses to bacterial antigens

    E. Memory B cells

Recently a patient was identified who had a defect in IL-1 receptor-associated kinase (IRAK)-dependent cellular signaling associated with her TLR4 receptor.

3. Which one of the following groups of pathogens would be expected to cause recurrent infections in this individual?

   A. Retroviruses, such as HIV-1

   B. Fungi that cause vaginal yeast infections

   C. Gram-negative bacteria

   D. Gastrointestinal viruses

   E. Insect-borne parasites

Anaerobic bacteria are often cultured from infected deep tissue abscesses.

4. If you were a neutrophil recruited to an anaerobic site to kill such a bacterium, which of the following substances would you most likely use?

   A. IL-12

   B. Nitric oxide

   C. Interferon-α

   D. Respiratory burst oxidase

   E. Cathelicidin

You are part of a research team that is attempting to design a better vaccine for the prevention of tuberculosis, which is caused by the intracellular bacterial pathogen *Mycobacterium tuberculosis*. One of your colleagues suggests that you include an adjuvant in the vaccine formulation.

5. Based on your knowledge of protective immunity to this pathogen, which one of the following would be a reasonable choice of an adjuvant component?

   A. A cytokine that promotes an IFN-γ response to mycobacterial antigens

   B. The complement peptide C3d, which will ensure adequate antibody production.

   C. Interleukin-10

   D. Bacterial lipopolysaccharide

   E. Lactoferrin

ANSWERS

1. The answer is C. Sepsis is a systemic inflammatory response to infection that results from exposure of the host to diverse microbial components expressing PAMP. With antibiotic treatment, large quantities of bacteria die and release these proinflammatory components, including bacterial LPS. The most important initial step is to discontinue antibiotic treatment until the septic episode has passed. Fluids are given to correct hypotension, and severe cases may need to be treated with pressors (eg, dopamine) to

maintain blood pressure. The patient's symptoms (hypotension, tachycardia, and hypoxia) are indicative of extreme vasodilation, the loss of fluid to the extravascular tissues, and inadequate tissue oxygenation. TNF-α is thought to be a major central mediator of systemic septic shock. The activation of complement would be expected to aggravate the systemic inflammatory response by further inducing vascular changes, hypotension, and hypoxia.

2. The correct answer is B. In a child of this age who has not previously been exposed to this bacterial pathogen or immunized against its antigens host defense is primarily mediated by the innate immune system. Neutrophils play a central role in clearing bacteria and recognize molecular patterns on these pathogens via their TLR. By contrast, T and B lymphocytes mediate adaptive immunity (eg, antibody formation), which requires several days to develop in an immunologically naive individual.

3. The correct answer is C. TLR4 is the signaling receptor for bacterial LPS, a component of the outer membrane of gram-negative bacteria. Patients with impaired TLR4 signaling are at risk for recurrent, life-threatening infections with gram-negative bacteria. TLR4 is not known to mediate protective responses to viruses, fungi, or parasites.

4. The correct answer is E. In the absence of molecular oxygen, neither reactive oxygen species (eg, superoxide) nor NO can be produced in sufficient quantities to kill bacteria. Under these conditions, the neutrophil must rely on oxygen-independent killing mechanisms, such as the action of its antimicrobial granule peptides.

5. The correct answer is A. Any cytokine that would promote the development of antigen-specific, IFN-γ-producing lymphocytes would probably have a favorable effect. Patients who cannot produce IFN-γ are at risk for developing mycobacterial infections. Interleukin-12 is a good example of an IFN-γ-inducing cytokine. Because this pathogen resides within tissue macrophages in chronically infected individuals, macrophage activation for intracellular killing is an essential protective response to infection.

CHAPTER 2
ADAPTIVE IMMUNITY

I. Adaptive immunity is distinguished by the following features.

A. Unlike innate immunity, **adaptive immunity** is an *acquired* response to antigen that is initiated by the recognition of discrete *antigenic determinants* on foreign invaders (Table 2–1).

B. The host is changed by its exposure to antigen; the individual becomes **"immunized"** against a particular antigen.

    1. The **primary response** to an antigen takes several days and requires antigen recognition, the activation and proliferation of T and B lymphocytes, and the differentiation of these cells into populations of **effector lymphocytes**.

    2. Sets of antigen-specific **memory T and B cells** are also generated that mediate **secondary responses** to the antigen at a later time.

    3. The long-term maintenance of memory and the return of lymphocytes to a nonactivated state are carefully controlled.

C. T and B lymphocytes are the primary mediators of adaptive immunity and recognize antigenic determinants by their cell surface **antigen receptors**.

    1. Receptors with specificity for **autoantigens** are expressed during the development of the adaptive immune system.

        a. Most lymphocytes with autoreactive receptors are deleted.

        b. Some autoreactive lymphocytes survive, but their activation is carefully controlled in the periphery.

    2. Whereas B cell receptors predominantly recognize soluble native antigens, T cell receptors recognize foreign antigens only on the surfaces of other host cells.

D. Many of the effector cells and molecules that mediate antigen clearance in adaptive immunity are the same as those that mediate protective innate immune responses.

II. Primary and secondary adaptive immune responses differ.

A. Evidence of a **primary immune response** to an antigen appears only after an initial **lag phase** (Figure 2–1).

B. Antibody produced following **active immunization** is **specific** for the immunizing antigen.

C. The host has enormous **diversity** in its capacity to respond to different antigens.

    1. Estimates of the number of different antigen receptors potentially expressed by B or T cells range from 10^8 to 10^9.

Table 2–1. Comparison of the properties of innate andadaptive immunity.

Property	Innate Immunity	Adaptive Immunity
Time	Immediate	Delayed
Recognition	Conserved, widely distributed microbial components	Discrete, diverse antigenic determinants Antigen presentation
Cells	Many cells: phagocytes, some lymphocytes, epithelial cells	Lymphocytes
Response	Uptake and clearance, danger signaling	Clearance, lysis, memory

    2. A diverse **immune repertoire** exists at birth in human beings and undergoes further changes based on the immunological experiences of the individual.

  D. Immunity mediated by lymphocytes or the antibodies they produce can be transferred from an immune host to a naive recipient.

    1. The transfer of antibodies is called **passive immunization**.

    2. The transfer of immune cells is called **adaptive immunization**.

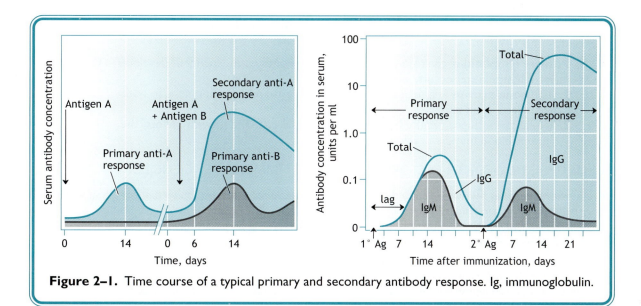

Figure 2–1. Time course of a typical primary and secondary antibody response. Ig, immunoglobulin.

NEWBORNS ACQUIRE MATERNAL IMMUNITY BY PASSIVE IMMUNIZATION

- *Newborns are passively immunized when their mothers transfer protective antibodies to them either across the placenta or through the colostrum and milk.*
- *The relative importance of these two routes in various mammalian species is determined by the structure of their placentas.*
- *Human beings have two cell layers separating fetal and maternal blood and actively transport maternal antibodies across the placenta.*
- *The class of antibody that is transported is immunoglobulin G (IgG) (Chapter 3) and it provides systemic antibody protection to the newborn.*
- *Colostral antibodies in humans are predominantly immunoglobulin A (IgA) and they protect the newborn intestinal tract from infectious pathogens.*
- *By contrast, the fetal calf receives no immunoglobulin from its mother during gestation, and is highly dependent upon suckling colostrum containing IgG antibodies during its first few days of life.*

   E. **Secondary responses** to an antigen in immune animals differ from primary adaptive immune responses (Figure 2–1).
   1. The lag period is shorter for the secondary response.
   2. The overall amount of antibody produced is greater in the secondary response.
   3. The class of antibody differs in the two responses.
      a. Primary antibody responses are mostly **immunoglobulin M (IgM)**.
      b. Secondary antibody responses consist primarily of non-IgM classes, especially **IgG**.
      c. The change that occurs in the class of antibody produced is called **isotype switching** and results in new functions being associated with the same antibody specificity (Chapter 3).
      d. The longer duration of the secondary response reflects the large number of memory B cells that are activated and the longer half-life of IgG in circulation compared to IgM.

III. Cells of the adaptive immune system are found in discrete lymphoid tissues and organs.

   A. **Primary lymphoid organs** are organs in which the antigen-independent development of lymphocytes occurs.
   1. The **bone marrow** is a major site of hematopoiesis and lymphopoiesis in both young and adult animals.
   2. Under the influence of the bone marrow stromal cells and growth factors, the various blood lineages develop.

HEMATOPOIETIC GROWTH FACTORS CAN CORRECT IMMUNE DEFICIENCIES

- **Cyclic neutropenia** *is a 3-week oscillating deficiency in the production of blood neutrophils that can leave patients at risk for infections (Table 2–2).*
- *The inherited form of the disease results from point mutations in the neutrophil elastase gene, suggesting that this protease participates in myelopoiesis.*
- *Treatment with* **colony-stimulating factor for granulocytes (CSF-G)** *replenishes neutrophil numbers in the blood during the neutropenic phase.*
- *By contrast,* **severe congenital neutropenia**, *which is due to a mutation in the gene for the receptor for CSF-G, is not responsive to CSF-G therapy.*

Table 2–2. Congenital leukocyte and lymphocyte deficiencies affecting immunity.

Cell Type	Subsets	Normal Cell Numbers (10^3 per μL) in the Blood of Adults	Congenital Deficiencies Affecting the Number of Cells in the Periphery
Leukocytes	Total	4–11	
	Neutrophils	2–7	Neonatal and cyclic neutropenia
	Monocytes	0.2–1.2	
Lymphocytes	Total	1.0–4.8	Severe combined immune deficiency
	B cells	0.1–0.7	X-linked agammaglobulinemia
	T cells	0.5–3.6	DiGeorge syndrome
	CD4$^+$ T cells	0.2–1.8	MHC class II deficiency
	CD8$^+$ T cells	0.1–0.9	MHC class I deficiency

- *Colony-stimulating factors for other hematopoietic progenitor cells, including erythropoietin and interleukin-3, have become standard treatments for many selective hematopoietic deficiencies.*

    3. Lymphocytes are also derived from a common self-renewing **hematopoietic stem cell** that gives rise to all blood cell lineages.

        a. In the appropriate inductive microenvironment, the pluripotent stem cell differentiates into a **lymphoid progenitor cell (LPC)**.

        b. The LPC can become a **progenitor T (pro-T) cell** or a **progenitor B (pro-B) cell**.

        c. In human beings, B lymphopoiesis occurs primarily in the bone marrow (Chapter 9), but T lymphocyte development moves to the thymus at the pro-T cell stage (Chapter 10).

        d. An important process that accompanies T and B cell differentiation in the bone marrow and thymus is the expression of surface antigen receptors.

DIGEORGE SYNDROME PATIENTS LACK A THYMUS

- *DiGeorge syndrome is a congenital condition arising from defective embryogenesis of the third and fourth pharyngeal pouches.*
- *Patients with DiGeorge syndrome show abnormalities in the structure of their major blood vessels, heart, and parathyroids and evidence thymic hypoplasia.*
- *Immunological abnormalities include severe lymphopenia (Table 2–2) at birth and early onset infections by opportunistic viruses and fungi.*
- *Antibody levels are normal at birth due to the transplacental passage of antibodies from the mother in utero.*
- *The immune deficiencies of these children can be cured by thymic transplantation from a suitable donor.*

    B. Secondary lymphoid organs are sites at which the host mounts adaptive immune responses to foreign invaders.

1. Secondary lymphoid organs and tissues include the spleen, lymph nodes, Peyer's patches, and widely distributed lymphoid follicles.

2. The **lymph node** is an encapsulated organ that receives antigens from subcutaneous and submucosal tissues via its **afferent lymphatics** (Figure 2–2).

   a. B cells are concentrated in discrete **primary and secondary follicles** within the cortex of lymph nodes, where they undergo antigen-driven differentiation.

   b. Memory B cells develop within the **germinal centers** of the cortex.

   c. T cells are located primarily in the **diffuse cortex** (or **paracortex**), where they associate with dendritic cells.

   d. Cells enter the lymph nodes in large numbers by crossing the high endothelial layer of **postcapillary venules** located in the diffuse cortex.

   e. Terminally differentiated B cells, called **plasma cells**, are found in the **medullary cords**, where they produce large amounts of antibody during their limited life-span.

   f. Secreted antibodies exit the lymph nodes via the **efferent lymphatics** and eventually enter the blood stream.

3. The **spleen** receives antigens through the blood circulation and contains areas functionally equivalent to those of the lymph nodes (Table 2–3).

4. Other important peripheral lymphoid tissues include the **Peyer's patches** and submucosa of the small intestine, which are sites in which mucosal antibody responses are induced (Chapter 9).

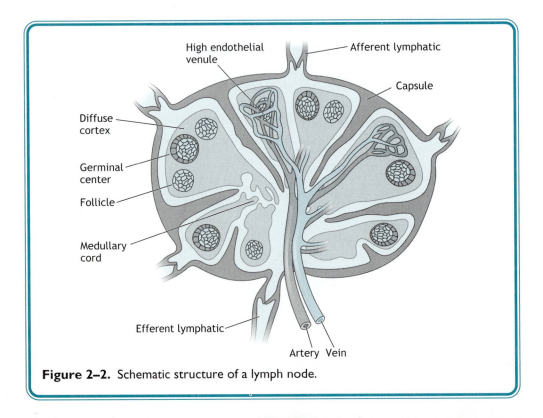

Figure 2–2. Schematic structure of a lymph node.

Table 2–3. Comparison of analogous structures in the lymph nodes and spleen.

Lymph Node	Spleen	Function
Follicles	Follicles	B cell activation and differentiation
Diffuse cortex	Periarteriolar lymphoid sheath	T cell activation and differentiation
Medullary cords	Red pulp cords	Antibody production by plasma cells
High endothelium of postcapillary venules	Marginal sinuses	Site of entry of lymphocytes from the recirulating lymphocyte pool
Afferent lymphatics	Marginal sinuses	Site of entry of antigens
Efferent lymphatics	Marginal sinuses	Point of exit of effector lymphocytes to join the recirculating pool

C. A **recirculating lymphocyte pool** of long-lived small lymphocytes continually travels between the various lymphoid tissues by a route that includes the blood and lymph (Figure 2–3).

1. Recirculating lymphocytes enter the lymph nodes from the blood by crossing the **high endothelial venules** in the diffuse cortex.
2. The cells exit the lymph nodes via the **efferent lymphatics** and migrate via the **common thoracic duct** to the blood stream.
3. Lymphocytes can exit the blood circulation by crossing the endothelium at many locations.

IV. The **clonal selection theory of adaptive immunity** proposes that an antigen selects and activates the appropriate clone of lymphocytes from a preformed diverse pool.

A. The theory predicts the following:
1. Each lymphocyte is precommitted to a particular antigen prior to encountering that antigen (Figure 2–4).
2. Lymphocytes recognize their antigens with cell surface antigen receptors.
3. The receptor on a given lymphocyte is specific for only one antigen.
4. Antigen binding to the receptor induces the expansion of a **clone** of cells, all with identical receptor specificity.
5. The antigen receptor on a given lymphocyte is uniform and identical to the antibody molecules secreted by the cell.

B. The theory has proven correct for both B and T lymphocytes with the following exceptions:
1. The B cell antigen receptor is actually a modified form of an antibody molecule (Chapter 4).
2. The T cell antigen receptor is not an antibody molecule (Chapter 6).
3. T cells do not secrete large amounts of their receptor molecules.

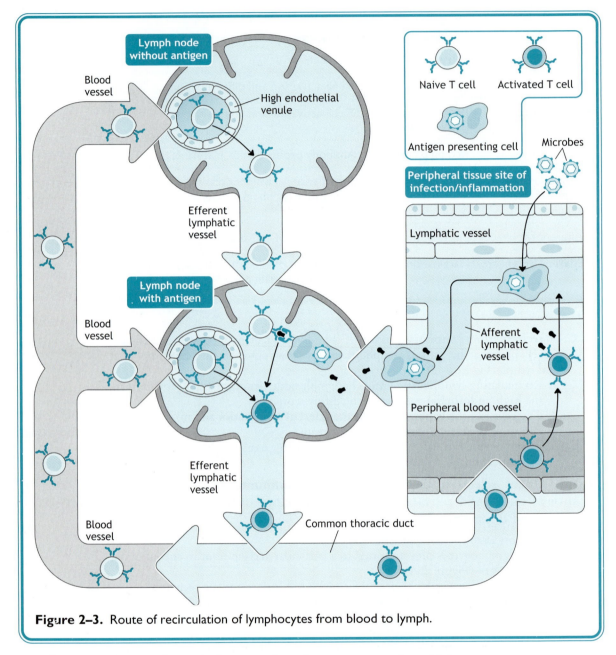

Figure 2–3. Route of recirculation of lymphocytes from blood to lymph.

C. The production of a pool of **memory lymphocytes** ensures that a higher concentration of specific antibody is produced in a more rapid fashion during a secondary response.

D. Because lymphocytes with receptors specific for autoantigens (**"forbidden clones"**) are mostly deleted or inactivated during their differentiation, **autoimmunity** is rare.

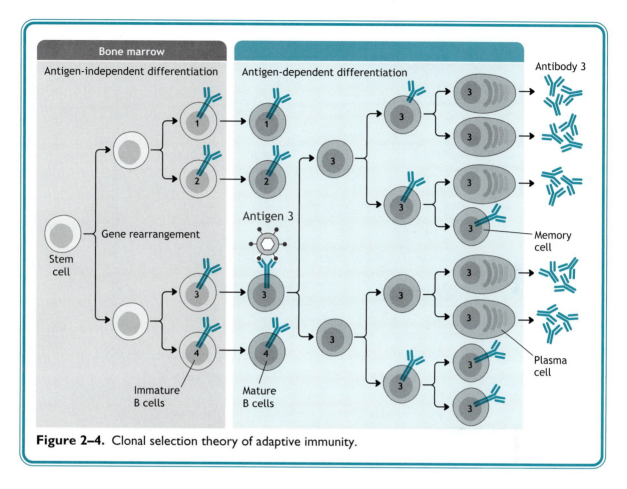

Figure 2–4. Clonal selection theory of adaptive immunity.

PERNICIOUS ANEMIA

- *Pernicious anemia (PA)* is an organ-specific autoimmune disease characterized by a decreased absorption of dietary vitamin B_{12}.
- Vitamin B_{12} is normally absorbed in the ileum as a complex with **intrinsic factor**, a protein synthesized by gastric parietal cells.
- Failure to absorb vitamin B_{12} in PA results from an autoimmune attack on gastric parietal cells and the clearance of intrinsic factor by autoantibodies.
- The resulting vitamin B_{12} deficiency results in impaired erythropoiesis (megaloblastic anemia).

V. Lymphocytes express antigen receptors.

  A. The **antigen receptor complexes** of T and B lymphocytes are similar in structure and function (Figure 2–5).

    1. The B cell receptor (BCR) for antigen consists of a membrane form of antibody and the accessory peptides **Igα** and **Igβ**.

      a. The BCR recognizes discrete antigenic determinants (epitopes) on soluble antigens.

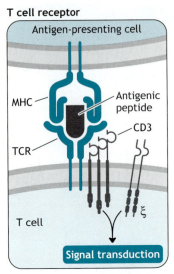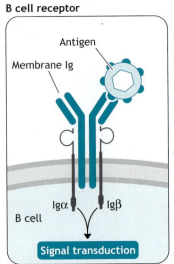

Figure 2–5. Antigen receptors on B and T lymphocytes. MHC, major histocompatibility complex; TCR, T cell receptor; Ig, immunoglobulin.

   B. Igα and Igβ mediate antigen-induced transmembrane signaling in B cells.
     1. The **T cell receptor (TCR)** complex consists of antibody-like peptides and signaling peptides.
       a. Unlike the BCR, the TCR can recognize only foreign antigens that are displayed on the surfaces of other cells.
         (1) T cells recognize surface-bound small peptides that are derived by proteolysis from native protein antigens.
         (2) The TCR recognizes determinants of the foreign peptide plus host cell surface molecules called **major histocompatibility complex (MHC) molecules**.
         (3) The cells on which these processed foreign peptides are displayed are collectively referred to as **antigen-presenting cells (APC)**.
       b. The MHC regulates antigen recognition by T cells.
         (1) Only peptides that can bind to the host's MHC molecules are recognized by T cells.
         (2) Two classes of MHC molecules control T cell antigen recognition in this fashion (Figure 2–6).
            (a) **MHC class I** is expressed on nearly all nucleated cells.
            (b) **MHC class II** is expressed on dendritic cells, macrophages, and B cells.
         (3) MHC restriction ensures that T cells will be activated by antigen only in proximity to other host cells.
            (a) **T helper (Th) cells** recognize antigen presented by MHC class II-expressing **dendritic cells (DC)**, B cells, and macrophages.

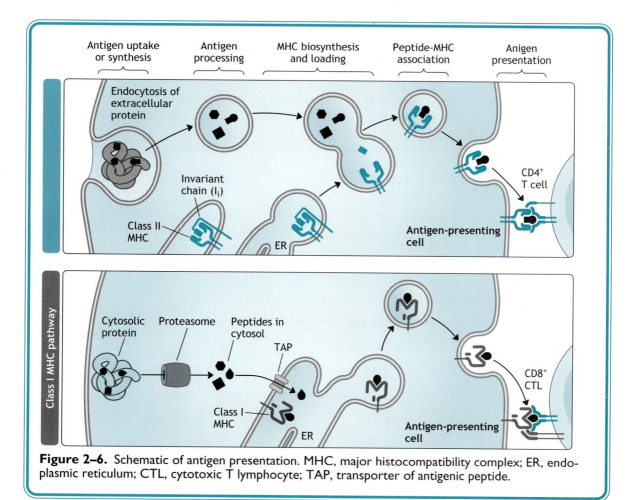

Figure 2–6. Schematic of antigen presentation. MHC, major histocompatibility complex; ER, endoplasmic reticulum; CTL, cytotoxic T lymphocyte; TAP, transporter of antigenic peptide.

  (b) **Cytotoxic T (Tc) cells** recognize antigen-expressing (eg, viral antigens), MHC class I-expressing host cells.

 c. The signaling peptides of the TCR are collectively referred to as **CD3**.

 d. The TCR complex is first expressed during T cell development in the thymus (Chapter 10).

T CELL DEFICIENCIES DUE TO ABNORMAL CD3 EXPRESSION

- *Mutations in two different CD3 peptides (CD3γ and CD3ε) have been described that decrease TCR expression.*
- *These patients show few peripheral T cells, susceptibility to viral and fungal infections, and autoimmunity.*
- *In addition to treatment for infections, these patients are candidates for hematopoietic stem cell transplantation, which can correct the defects.*
- *This and other congenital immune deficiencies are described in detail at the Online Mendelian Inheritance in Man web site maintained by the National Library of Medicine (www.ncbi.nlm.nih.gov/omim).*

C. **Antigen presentation** requires the processing and MHC-dependent display of antigenic determinants (Figure 2–6).

1. Any nucleated cell can potentially present peptide antigens through MHC class I.
   a. T cells that recognize peptides + MHC class I bear a distinguishing cell surface coreceptor called **CD8**.
   b. Most CD8+ T cells are cytotoxic.
2. DC, B cells, monocytes, and macrophages express MHC class II and can present antigenic peptides via class II molecules.
   a. T cells that recognize peptides + MHC class II bear a distinguishing cell surface coreceptor called **CD4**.
   b. Most CD4+ T cells secrete cytokines that regulate the activation of other immune cells.

VI. Lymphocytes bear a number of additional cell surface molecules that control their activation, migration, or effector functions.

Table 2–4. Properties of CD markers.[a]

CD Category	Examples	Expression	Major Functions
Antigen presentation	CD1	Dendritic cells	Presents glycolipid antigens
Adhesion molecules	CD18	Leukocytes	Adhesion to endothelium
Coreceptors	CD4	T cells	Coactivates with TCR-CD3
Cytokine receptors	CD25	B cells	Binding of IL-2
Ig-binding receptors	CD32	Macrophages	Binding IgG–antigen complexes
Signal transduction	CD3	T cells	Mediates signaling of TCR
Homing receptors	CD62L	B and T cells	Homing to lymph nodes
Death-inducing receptors	CD120	Many cells	TNF-α-induced apoptosis
Enzymes	CD45	T cells	Phosphatase; regulates TCR signaling
Complement receptors	CD55	Many cells	Regulates complement activation
Blood group markers	CD240D	Erythrocytes	Major Rh antigen

[a]For a more complete list of CD markers, see Appendix I. TCR, T cell receptor; IL-2, interleukin 2; IgG, immunoglobulin G; TNF, tumor necrosis factor.

A. **Coreceptors** on lymphocytes promote signaling through the TCR and BCR.
   1. Coreceptors lower the threshold for lymphocyte activation through their antigen receptors.
   2. Coreceptors can act by modulating intracellular signaling pathways or increasing the expression of other receptors.
B. T and B cells express a range of **cytokine receptors** that provides additional signals for cell activation.
C. Receptors that bind **IgG molecules** present in antigen–antibody complexes (**Fc receptors**) typically inhibit B cell activation.
D. **Cell adhesion molecules** mediate lymphocyte migration between and within tissues and increase the binding between lymphocyte subsets.
E. One method for cataloging cell surface molecules is the **cluster of differentiation (CD)** scheme that assigns a CD number to each unique cell surface molecule (Table 2–4, Appendix I, and www.hlda8.org/).

PHENOTYPING OF LYMPHOCYTE SUBSETS

- *Human lymphocyte subsets are routinely enumerated in the clinical laboratory by a technique known as **flow cytometry** (Chapter 5).*
- *Monoclonal antibodies to the **CD markers** of interest (Table 2–4) are labeled with a fluorochrome and used to stain cells.*
- *The flow cytometer detects labeled antibody binding to the cell and thereby enumerates surface CD molecules on blood cells or cells prepared from solid tissues (eg, tumors).*
- *Abnormal lymphocyte numbers are associated with congenital or acquired immune deficiencies, infections, and neoplastic conditions.*
- *Leukemias and lymphomas can be typed and staged by defining the CD markers they express.*

CLINICAL PROBLEMS

A 2-month-old male child presents with thrush (a yeast infection in the oral cavity), diarrhea, and failure to thrive. His complete blood count reveals a severe lymphopenia. Flow cytometry demonstrates a very low number of CD3⁺ lymphocytes in his blood, but normal numbers of membrane IgM⁺ lymphocytes when compared to age-matched controls.

1. Which one of the following represents the most likely underlying disease in this child?
   A. X-linked agammaglobulinemia (XLA)
   B. DiGeorge syndrome
   C. Neonatal neutropenia
   D. Myeloperoxidase deficiency
   E. Aplastic anemia

A patient has a history of recurrent pneumonias that reappear within a week following completion of antibiotic therapy. She is found to have a deficiency in the expression of CD18.

2. Which of the following two clinical abnormalities would you most expect to find in such a patient? More than one answer may be correct.

A. Lymphopenia

B. Leukocytosis

C. Recurrent viral infections

D. Recurrent bacterial infections

E. Abnormal BCR cell signaling

F. Agammaglobulinemia

G. Reduced T lymphocyte receptor expression

3. Which of the following is a "pattern recognition receptor"?

A. BCR

B. Interleukin-1 receptor

C. Fc receptor

D. CD4

E. Mannose receptor

A patient presents with a lymphocytosis and enlarged lymph nodes, and a biopsy of the bone marrow is performed. Ninety percent of the patient's bone marrow cells stain with a fluorescent antibody specific for CD3.

4. Which of the following is a reasonable differential diagnosis?

A. AIDS

B. DiGeorge syndrome

C. T cell leukemia

D. Cytomegalovirus infection

E. This is a normal laboratory finding.

Patients with deficiencies in antibody production can often present with the same types of infections as are seen in patients with phagocytic cell deficiencies.

5. Which of the following statements **best explains** this observation?

A. Autoantibodies can remove phagocytic cells from the blood circulation.

B. Plasma cells are the direct progenitors of certain phagocytic cells.

C. Macrophages can differentiate into antibody-producing plasma cells.

D. Antibodies are important opsonins that promote microbe recognition by phagocytes.

E. Antibodies are essential for the continued production of phagocytic cells by the bone marrow.

ANSWERS

1. The correct answer is B. The finding of low lymphocyte counts in the blood (lymphopenia) affecting only T cells suggests a deficiency in cell-mediated immunity secondary to decreased T cell numbers, such as in thymic dysplasia (DiGeorge syndrome). This would be expected to lead to opportunistic infections by intracellular pathogens, such as the yeast *Candida albicans*.

2. The correct answers are B and D. The CD18 gene encodes for an adhesion molecule, and patients with decreased CD18 expression show poor leukocyte adhesion to the vascular endothelium. The increase in leukocyte production seen during infections results in an increased number of leukocytes in the blood (leukocytosis). The resulting decreased leukocyte migration to infection sites impairs clearance of extracellular bacterial pathogens.

3. The correct answer is E. The mannose receptor recognizes the spatial arrangement of mannose residues that is found only on microbial surfaces.

4. The correct answer is C. Finding large numbers of CD3⁺ cells in the bone marrow is most likely indicative of neoplastic T cells (leukemia), because CD3 is normally expressed only after the pro-T cell migrates to the thymus.

5. The answer is D. Antibodies of certain classes can bind to microbial surface antigens and mark them for uptake by phagocytic cells. This is because phagocytes bear opsonic receptors that bind antibody-coated particles and signal an increased rate of uptake. Thus, patients who lack certain antibodies will show diminished phagocytic cell function due to impaired opsonophagocytosis.

CHAPTER 3
ANTIGENS
AND ANTIBODIES

I. Antigens

A. An **antigen** is a substance that can elicit an adaptive immune response.

B. Most natural and medically important antigens are macromolecules or substances that can bind covalently to them.

C. Naturally occurring antigens include proteins, polysaccharides, lipids, and nucleic acids.

D. The region of an antigen that is recognized by the immune system is called an **antigenic determinant** or **epitope**.

E. Antigens generally have two properties.

  1. Immunogenicity is the capacity to induce an immune response.

    a. Immunogenicity is determined by the molecular mass, molecular complexity (number of potential determinants), and conformation of an antigen.

    b. A high degree of phylogenetic disparity between an antigen and the host generally promotes immunogenicity.

  2. Antigenicity is the ability to bind specifically to antibody molecules or antigen receptors on lymphocytes.

  3. A **hapten** is a molecule that is antigenic, but not immunogenic.

    a. A hapten generally has a molecular mass of less than 10,000 Da.

    b. A hapten can become immunogenic if it is covalently attached (conjugated) to a **carrier molecule**.

    c. Some haptens can cause **allergic dermatitis** if they bind to proteins in the skin.

    d. Conjugating microbial epitopes (haptens) to carrier proteins is an effective approach to producing highly immunogenic vaccines.

PENICILLIN IS A HAPTEN THAT CAN INDUCE IMMUNE-MEDIATED TISSUE DAMAGE

- *Penicillin G is a small drug (MW 356) that can bind to a variety of host proteins, including those on the surface of human erythrocytes.*
- *Antipenicillin antibodies can be produced that cause **autoimmune hemolytic anemia**.*
- *The **Coombs test** is used to determine if an anemia has an immune basis by determining whether immunoglobulin G (IgG) antibodies are present on the patient's erythrocytes.*
- *The treatment of Coombs-positive anemias includes discontinuing the drug (hapten) and transfusing normal ABO-matched erythrocytes.*

F. Antigenic determinants that bind to antibodies and B cell antigen receptors are often different from those that bind to T cell antigen receptors (Table 3–1).
   1. Determinants recognized by antibodies or B cells are typically found on the exposed **hydrophilic** surface of an antigen molecule.
   2. Antigens that bind to the T cell antigen receptor typically do not possess their native conformation.
      a. Most antigens that stimulate T cells are proteins.
      b. For a protein to be recognized by a T cell it must be degraded into peptides and presented by an antigen-presenting cell (APC).
      c. T cell determinants are not limited to surface exposed regions of proteins and can be derived from internal hydrophobic protein domains.

II. Antibodies

   A. All antibodies are **immunoglobulins (Igs)**.

   B. Igs are a homologous family of proteins with considerable structural heterogeneity.

   C. Most Igs migrate in the "gamma" region upon **serum protein electrophoresis** and are therefore called γ-**globulins** (Figure 3–1).

INTRAVENOUS IMMUNOGLOBULIN (IVIG)

CLINICAL CORRELATION

- *Immunoglobulins (γ-globulins) are routinely given to patients for the prevention or treatment of various diseases.*
- *IVIGs are often used to treat congenital antibody deficiencies and must be given repeatedly.*
- *Because IVIG is greater than 95% IgG, its primary immune benefit in immunodeficient patients is to provide protection against extracellular microbial pathogens or their toxic products.*
- *Some infectious diseases in normal individuals, such as rabies and hepatitis, can be effectively prevented with γ-globulins prepared from specific immune donors that are administered shortly after a suspected infection.*

   D. The structure of antibodies was first determined by studying Igs purified from the sera of patients with **multiple myeloma**.

Table 3–1. Comparison of the antigenic determinants recognized by B and T lymphocytes.

Property	B cells	T cells
Conformation dependent	+	−
Hydrophillic/hydrophobic	Hydrophillic	Hydrophillic and hydrophobic
Location of determinants	Surface	Surface and internal
MHC dependent	−	+
Examples	Native proteins and carbohydrates	Peptides

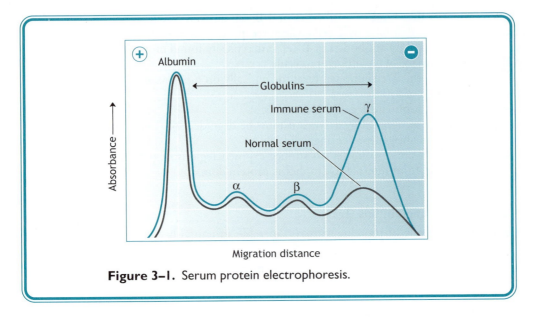

Figure 3–1. Serum protein electrophoresis.

1. Multiple myeloma is a malignancy of a clone of Ig-producing plasma cells.
2. Myeloma Igs (also called **M proteins**) are monoclonal and structurally homogeneous.
3. All M proteins belong to one of five structurally distinct Ig **classes** or **isotypes**.
4. The most frequently encountered isotype among myeloma proteins is IgG.
   a. IgG molecules have the molecular formula H_2L_2 and show **bilateral symmetry** (Figure 3–2).
      (1) Each IgG molecule contains two identical **heavy (H) chains**.
      (2) The H chains of IgG molecules are designated γ chains and have a molecular mass of approximately 50,000 Da.
      (3) H chains are linked to one another by *inter*-chain disulfide bonds.
      (4) Each IgG molecule contains two identical **light (L) chains**, each with a molecular mass of approximately 25,000 Da.
      (5) L chains are covalently linked to H chains by *inter*-chain disulfide bonds.
   b. *Intra*-chain disulfide bonds in both H and L chains maintain protein folds that define **Ig domains** of approximately 110 amino acids in length (Figure 3–2).
   c. There are two such domains in L chains and four in γ H chains.
5. There are a total of five **classes or isotypes** of human Ig, designated IgG, IgM, IgA, IgE, and IgD (Table 3–2).
   a. Each Ig has the core molecular H_2L_2 structure and contains H chains unique to that isotype.
   b. IgG, IgM, IgA, IgE, and IgD have γ, μ, α, ε, and δ, H chains, respectively.
      (1) γ, α, and δ chains have molecular masses of 50,000–60,000 Da.
      (2) μ and ε chains, which have an additional Ig domain, have molecular masses of 65,000–70,000 Da (Table 3–2).

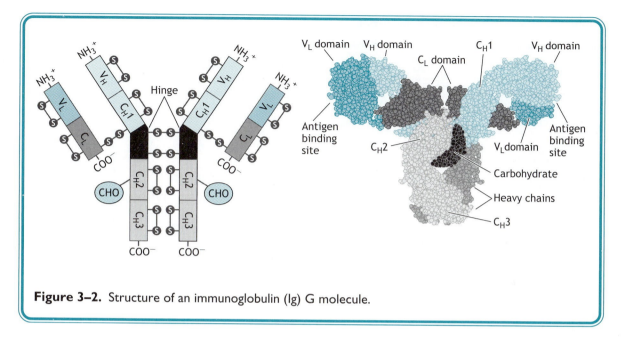

Figure 3–2. Structure of an immunoglobulin (Ig) G molecule.

    c. The IgG class is further subdivided into the IgG_1, IgG_2, IgG_3, and IgG_4 subclasses.

    d. The IgA class is further subdivided into the IgA_1 and IgA_2 subclasses.

  6. All Igs can occur in two forms, secreted and membrane bound.

  7. There are two human L chain **types**, termed κ and λ.

    a. In any one immunoglobulin molecule, both L chains are either κ or λ.

    b. The overall κ:λ ratio for the Igs found in human serum is approximately 60:40.

  8. Oligosaccharides are covalently attached to the carboxyl-terminal half of H chains, especially within μ and ε chains.

MULTIPLE MYELOMA

- *Patients with multiple myeloma can have extremely high levels of Igs in their plasma that are often first detected by serum protein electrophoresis (Figure 3–1).*
- *Because their cancers are monoclonal and have a homogeneous charge, the abnormal M protein appears on electrophoresis as a "spike."*
- *Each M protein has a single H chain class and a single L chain type.*
- *Many patients with myeloma also have high concentrations of Ig L chains in their urine, which are produced in excess by their myeloma cells.*
- *In a given patient, these **Bence–Jones proteins** are monoclonal, dimeric, and either κ or λ, but not both.*
- *Finding a significant departure from the normal 60:40 κ:λ ratio in serum or urinary L chains is diagnostic of a **monoclonal gammopathy**, such as myeloma.*

  E. IgM and IgA molecules can exist as multimers (Figure 3–3).

    1. Serum IgM is a pentamer of the core H_2L_2 structure that is joined together by intersubunit disulfide bonds and stabilized by a 15-kDa **joiner (J) chain**.

Table 3–2. Properties of human immunoglobulin isotypes.

Property	IgG	IgM	IgA	IgE	IgD
Subclasses	IgG$_{1-4}$	None	IgA$_{1-2}$	None	None
Heavy chain	γ	μ	α	ε	δ
C$_H$ domains	3	4	3	4	3
L chain	κ or λ	κ or λ	κ or λ	κ or λ	κ or λ
Molecular mass[a] (secreted form)	150,000	900,000	150,000 570,000[b]	190,000	170,000
Serum concentration (mg/dL)	1350	150	300	0.05	3
Serum half-life (days)	23	5	6	2	3
Activates complement (classical pathway)	+	++	–	–	–
Placental transport	+	–	–	–	–
Mucosal epithelial transport	–	+	++	–	–
Mast cell degranulation	–	–	–	+	–
Binding to phagocyte Fc receptors	+	–[c]	–	–	–
Binding to Fc receptors on natural killer cells	+	–	–	–	–
Antigen receptor of naive B cells	–	+	–	–	+

[a]Refers to the predominant forms in serum and external secretions, not the form found on B cell surfaces.
[b]Secretory IgA found in external secretions is a dimer with an associated J chain and secretory component.
[c]Recent evidence suggests Fc$_\mu$ receptors on neutrophils may mediate host defense against spirochetes.

    2. Serum IgA is primarily a monomer, but secretory IgA that is found in external secretions (eg, saliva and colostrum) is dimeric and contains a J chain polypeptide.

      a. Dimeric IgA is synthesized in the intestinal submucosa and efficiently translocated across the mucosal epithelium.

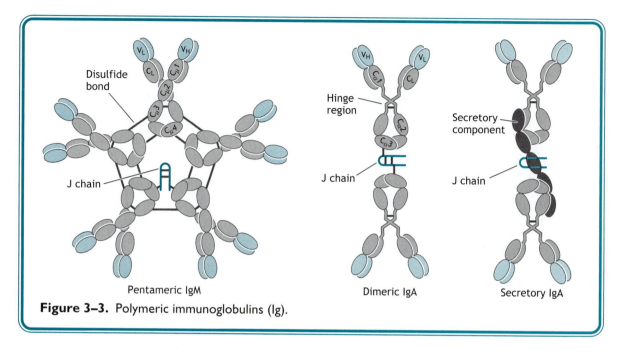

Figure 3–3. Polymeric immunoglobulins (Ig).

    b. During the process of translocation, epithelial cells add a 70-kDa peptide, called a **secretory component (SC)**, to the IgA molecule (Figure 3–3).
    (1) SC protects secretory IgA from proteolytic digestion.
    (2) SC promotes the binding of secretory IgA to the mucous layer of the epithelium.

F. Amino acid sequencing of myeloma H and L chains shows that they have constant (C) and variable (V) regions.
    1. The amino-terminal half of an L chain is designated the **variable light (V_L) domain.**
        a. Amino acid sequence diversity in V_L domains is greatest within the three **hypervariable regions**, HV1, HV2, and HV3.
        b. HV regions are also called **complementarity determining regions (CDR)**, because they comprise the walls of the antigen-binding cleft.
    2. The carboxyl-terminal half of an L chain is relatively constant and is designated as the **constant light (C_L)** domain (C_κ or C_λ).
    3. As with V_L domains, the amino-terminal V_H domains of H chains are highly variable when several H chains are compared.
        a. V_H domains contain three hypervariable regions.
        b. V_H domains that have different amino acid sequences generally have different specificities.
    4. The antigen-binding activity of an Ig depends on both its V_H and V_L domains.
    5. The three carboxyl-terminal C_H domains of IgG H chains are designated C_H1, C_H2, and C_H3.

G. Structure and function in Igs are related.
    1. The distribution of Ig function within Ig domains was first revealed by studying proteolytic fragments of the molecules.

2. Enzymatic digestion of rabbit IgG antibodies with the protease **papain** yields three fragments.
   a. Two are identical **antigen-binding fragments (Fab)** consisting of the V_H + C_H1 domains.
   b. Each Fab can bind one molecule of antigen.
   c. One **Fc fragment** is also generated and consists of the carboxyl-terminal half of the two disulfide-linked H chains (ie, the C_H2 + C_H3 domains in IgG).
   d. The Fc region mediates the opsonic activity of IgG antibodies by binding them to **Fc receptors** on phagocytic cells.
3. The **effector functions** of antibodies depend on the structures of their C_H domains.
   a. Many functions of antibodies are not expressed until they have bound their antigens, which induces conformational changes in the C_H domains.
   b. Transplacental transport, transepithelial transport, and mast cell binding of Igs do not require prior binding of the Ig to its antigen.
   c. A **hinge region** in many C_H domains is responsible for the flexibility in antibody conformation necessary for cooperative antigen binding.
4. The principal functions of IgG antibodies are to serve as opsonins, activate the complement system, provide fetal protection following transplacental transport, and inhibit B cell activation (Table 3–2).
5. The principal functions of IgM antibodies are to serve as antigen receptors on naive B cells, activate the complement system, clear circulating antigen, and provide host defense at mucosal surfaces.
6. The principal function of IgA antibodies is to provide antibody defense at mucosal surfaces.
7. The principal function of IgE antibodies is to mediate allergic reactions by promoting mast cell degranulation.
8. The principal function of IgD antibodies is to serve as an antigen receptor on naive B cells.

ISOTYPE SWITCHING AND CONJUGATE VACCINES

- *Antibody production undergoes **isotype switching** late in the primary adaptive immune response (Chapter 2).*
- *This associates new antibody functions with the same antibody specificity, a principle illustrated by the Haemophilus influenzae type b (Hib) conjugate vaccine.*
- *Hib is one of the leading causes of bacterial nasopharyngeal infections in children and can progress to pneumonia and life-treatening meningitis.*
- *Immune elimination of H influenzae requires antibodies to the polysaccharide capsule of this organism.*
- *H influenzae capsular polysaccharide vaccines have not proven effective at eliciting opsonic IgG antibodies in children.*
- *By contrast, the conjugate vaccine consisting of Hib capsular polysaccharides covalently linked to a foreign carrier protein (eg, the tetanus toxoid vaccine protein) is quite effective at inducing protective IgG antibodies in children.*
- *A description of the Hib conjugate vaccine and other recommended pediatric vaccines can be found at www.cdc.gov/nip/recs/child-schedule.pdf.*

H. **Natural antibodies** appear early in life.
   1. Most natural antibodies belong to the **IgM class** of Igs.

2. Many natural antibodies are produced in response to carbohydrate antigens present on microbial flora.
3. Some natural antibodies also cross-react with carbohydrate structures on host cells.
   a. The **isohemagglutinins**, natural antibodies to the **ABO blood group antigens**, can mediate the destruction of transfused mismatched blood.
   b. Isohemagglutinins recognize the terminal sugar groups of the ABO polysaccharide antigens expressed by erythrocytes and endothelial cells (Figure 3–4).
      (1) Three blood group antigens are defined by this sytem: A, B, and H.
      (2) Because the ABO genes are expressed in a codominant fashion, the potential ABO types are A, B, AB, and O.
      (3) Individuals produce isohemagglutinins specific for the ABO antigens that they lack (Table 3–3).
      (4) With regard to blood transfusions, the **universal donor** is type O, because this individual lacks antigens that would be recognized by ABO-incompatible recipients.
      (5) The **universal recipient** is type AB, because this individual lacks antibodies that would destroy ABO-incompatible donor erythrocytes.
   c. Natural antibodies can also mediate the rejection of **xenotransplants**, organs exchanged between species (Chapter 17).

III. Additional Ig heterogeneity

A. Slight sequence variations can exist between immunoglobulin molecules of the same isotype (eg, IgG_1) from different individuals.
   1. These inherited genetic markers reside within the C_H or C_L domains of human Igs and are called **allotypes**.
   2. Antiallotype antibodies are sometimes produced following pregnancy, blood transfusions, or γ-globulin therapy.

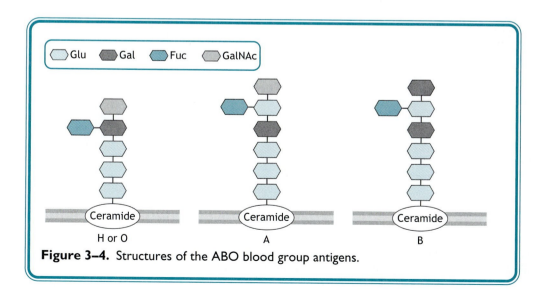

Figure 3–4. Structures of the ABO blood group antigens.

Table 3–3. Antigens and antibodies of the ABO blood group system.

Blood Group Type	Genotypes	Antigens	Isohemagglutinins
A	AA, AO	A	Anti-B
B	BB, BO	B	Anti-A
AB	AB	A and B	None
O	OO	H	Anti-A and anti-B

B. Igs of the same isotype can also be distinguished from one another by their V regions.

   1. An antibody of a given specificity has unique $V_L + V_H$ domains, the combination of which specifies its **idiotype**.

   2. An antibody molecule and the B cell receptor of the clone of B cells that produced it have the same idiotype (Chapter 2).

   3. Antiidiotype antibodies can block the binding of antigen to its antibody.

IV. Monoclonal Igs

A. Monoclonal antibodies are only rarely produced in response to active immunization with natural antigens.

B. In abnormal conditions called **monoclonal gammopathies** a single clone of B cells or plasma cells produces a monoclonal Ig.

   1. Malignant monoclonal gammopathies include **multiple myeloma, non-Hodgkin's lymphoma**, and **Waldenström's macroglobulinemia**.

   2. Benign monoclonal gammopathies include **light chain disease** and **monoclonal gammopathy of undetermined significance (MGUS)**, a condition that is common in the elderly.

   3. **Bence–Jones proteins** are monoclonal Ig L chains that are found in the urine.

      a. The exclusion properties of the renal glomeruli permit passage of L chains, but not H chains.

      b. These Bence–Jones proteins can accumulate in renal tubular epithelial cells, where they can cause necrosis.

ABNORMAL IG SYNTHESIS AND CRYOPATHIES

- *The excess production of Ig L chains can result in a number of systemic effects, including **cryoglobulinemia**, the microprecipitation of circulating proteins in the cold.*
- *Complications of cryoglobulinemia involving Ig proteins include cyanosis of the digits, hemorrhage, thrombosis, and gangrene.*
- *In B cell malignancies, cryoglobulins are monoclonal and can include intact M components or free L chains.*
- *In addition to treatment of the primary disease (eg, myeloma), plasma exchange and **cryophoresis** (reinfusion of autologous plasma following removal of the cryoglobulins) have met with some success.*

C. **Hybridoma antibody technology** allows production of a monoclonal antibody with a desired specificity.
1. Hybridomas are produced by fusing a nonsecreting myeloma cell with B cells from an animal that has been immunized with an antigen of interest.
2. Monoclonal antibody-producing hybridomas with the desired specificity are then identified, selected, and expanded in cell culture.
3. Hybridoma antibodies show less cross-reactivity than conventional antisera and are preferred for diagnostic tests (Chapter 5).

NOVEL ANTIBODY-MEDIATED THERAPIES

- *Immunotoxins* are conjugates composed of lethal plant or microbial toxins covalently linked to antibodies that target the conjugate to specific cells or tissues (eg, leukemia cells).
- *Bispecific antibodies* are genetically engineered to contain Fab regions specific for two different antigens (eg, CD3 on T cells and a tumor target antigen).
- *Humanized mouse hybridoma antibodies* are genetically engineered to contain mouse Ig hypervariable regions embedded in a human IgG antibody framework.
- This minimizes the likelihood that the host will mount an immune response to the foreign mouse hybridoma antibody sequences.
- *Fusion proteins* produced by covalently linking cytokine receptor domains to Ig molecules have extended half-lives in circulation and have proven effective for the treatment of cytokine-mediated inflammatory diseases.

CLINICAL PROBLEMS

You are considering treatment options for a 1-year-old child with a congenital immune deficiency. He has very low serum IgG levels and recurrent bacterial infections, and he lacks B cells in his peripheral lymph nodes. You decide to treat with IVIGs, which you realize may be required throughout his life.

1. How often will you have to administer IVIG to maintain a consistent level of protective immunity in this child?
   A. Twice per week
   B. Once per week
   C. Once every 3 weeks
   D. Once every 6 months
   E. Yearly

A child is immunized by the intramuscular route at 2, 4, and 6 months of age with tetanus toxoid, a protein antigen. One week following each immunization her serum is collected and analyzed for antitoxoid antibodies.

2. Which of the following properties would characterize the serum collected after the third immunization compared to that collected after the first immunization?

A. Increased specificity for tetanus toxoid

B. Increased ability of the serum to promote the uptake of the toxoid by phagocytic cells

C. Increased complement activation by antigen–antibody complexes formed with the serum

D. Increased reactivity with autoantigens of the host

E. Decreased binding of the toxoid

An 80-year-old man presents with slight pain on urination, and his physician orders a test for protein in his urine. An elevated urinary protein level prompts the physician to request a urine protein electrophoresis, which shows a protein spike.

3. Which of the following additional findings would be most consistent with a diagnosis of a benign monoclonal gammopathy?

A. A high concentration of serum IgG and elevated β and γ region proteins on protein electrophoresis

B. Elevated concentrations of κ and λ L chains in his serum

C. A high κ:λ ratio (100:1) among his urinary L chains

D. An elevated erythrocyte sedimentation rate

E. Recurrent bacterial infections

Johnny is a 3-month-old infant in need of a blood transfusion. The blood bank has determined that Johnny's parents are both blood group type AB.

4. Which of the following findings would indicate that Johnny has an ABO type different from that of his parents?

A. His serum reacts with type O erythrocytes.

B. His cells react with anti-A.

C. His cells react with both anti-A and anti-B.

D. His serum reacts with his father's cells.

E. His cells react with his mother's serum.

A researcher has produced an idiotype-specific antibody by immunizing a rabbit with an M protein purified from the serum of a myeloma patient. This antibody does not react with any other M protein tested.

5. With which of the following structures would this antibody react?

A. Fab fragment

B. J chain

C. C_H1 domain

D. Fc fragment

E. Fc receptor binding site

ANSWERS

1. The correct answer is C. IVIG is a γ-globulin preparation derived from pooled immune donor plasma and contains primarily IgG, which is what this patient lacks. The half-life of human IgG in the circulation is 23 days (approximately 3 weeks).

2. The correct answer is B. One of the principal reasons for repeated immunizations is to induce Ig class switching (eg, a change from predominantly IgM to predominantly IgG production). This has the effect of introducing new functions associated with the additional isotypes. For example, IgG (but not IgM) is a potent opsonin due to the presence of Fc receptors on phagocytic cells that recognize γ heavy chains.

3. The correct answer is C. To diagnose a monoclonal gammopathy the clinical laboratory must demonstrate a predominance of one L chain (κ or λ) over the other, which would alter the normal 60:40 ratio. Monoclonal gammopathies appear on electrophoresis as a "spike," whereas polyclonal gammopathies appear as an elevated amount of protein across a wide electrophoretic range (ie, the entire γ region). Monoclonal gammopathy of undetermined significance is a common finding in patients in this particular age group.

4. The correct answer is D. Johnny could theoretically be either A, B, or AB. If his serum reacts with his father's cells, he must have either anti-A or anti-B in his serum. Either finding would indicate he has a blood type that is different from his parents, because AB individuals have no antibodies to ABO antigens.

5. The correct answer is A. If this antibody is indeed specific for only this patient's M protein, it must be recognizing the V region of the Ig. The only structure listed that contains V region domains is the Fab fragment.

CHAPTER 4
IMMUNOGLOBULIN GENE EXPRESSION

I. A fundamental problem posed by the unusual structure of immunoglobulin (Ig) molecules is solved by a novel genetic mechanism.

    A. Igs are unusual in that millions of different V region sequences exist among the pool of Ig polypeptide chains.

    B. These diverse V regions are found within polypeptides that show limited diversity in their C region sequences.

    C. The germ line genome of a species is not large enough to encode all of the potential Ig V region sequences.

    D. To form the pool of Ig V region sequences a limited number of inherited **Ig gene segments** undergoes genetic recombination and random reassortment.

        1. The genetic capacity to generate the diverse family of Ig proteins exists within the germ line of every cell.

        2. Rearrangements of Ig DNA by somatic recombination occurs only in B cells and is a random pretranscriptional process.

        3. Diversity is generated prior to exposure to foreign antigen.

        4. Each member of the species has a similar **potential repertoire** of Igs.

II. Ig genes are initially organized in a germ line configuration.

    A. There are three **gene families** (also referred to as **loci**) that encode Ig polypeptides, the κ, λ, and H chain gene families.

        1. There are only 10–100 **gene segments** at each locus.

        2. Both the κ and λ chain loci contain **constant (C), variable (V),** and **joiner (J) gene segments** (Figure 4–1).

        3. The H chain locus has a similar arrangement with a 5′ cluster of V_H gene segments, several J_H segments, a group of **diversity (D_H)** segments (not seen in the L chain loci), and nine C_H segments.

            a. The C_H gene segments correspond to the nine classes and subclasses of human H chains.

            b. Each of the C_H segments consists of a cluster of three or four exons encoding the different C_H domains of secreted Ig H chains (Figure 3–2).

            c. One or two short exons follow these C_H exon clusters that code the transmembrane and cytoplasmic regions of membrane H chains.

        4. Latent promoters are found upstream of each V_κ, V_λ, and V_H segment.

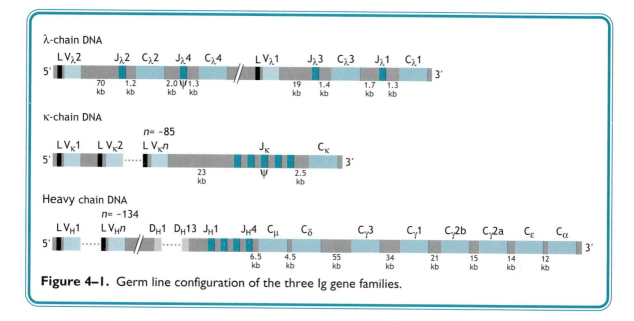

Figure 4–1. Germ line configuration of the three Ig gene families.

Ig LOCUS DELETIONS

- *Deletion mutations affecting large regions of the human Ig loci are known to exist.*
- *Among a consanguineous population of Tunisians, several individuals with homozygous deletions in the H chain locus have been identified.*
- *One haplotype has a multigene deletion of the entire $C_\gamma 1$-to-C_ε segment (Figure 4–1).*
- *An affected individual showed normal numbers of B cells in his peripheral lymphoid tissues, but his serum contained no detectable IgG_1, IgG_2, IgG_4, or IgA_1.*
- *In some instances of Ig locus deletions one Ig class can apparently compensate for the absence of another, thus preventing any increased susceptibility to infection.*

III. The recombination of Ig gene segments precedes the expression of a complete Ig gene.

  A. Somatic recombination rearranges the order of the various segments within the L chain loci to create a functional Ig gene.

  B. Recombination generates diversity within the V regions of L chain polypeptides.

   1. For example, recombination at the κ locus brings one V_κ segment, one J_κ segment, and one C_κ segment into proximity with one another (Figure 4–2).

   2. Recombination involves the cleavage of double-stranded DNA and its religation.

   3. A **V(D)J recombinase** catalyzes cleavage and is expressed only in lymphocytes.

   a. V(D)J recombinase consists of two components encoded by **recombination activating gene 1 (*Rag1*)** and **recombination activating gene 2 (*Rag2*)**.

   b. Mutations within *Rag1* or *Rag2* prevent the rearrangement of the Ig and T cell receptor (TCR) loci.

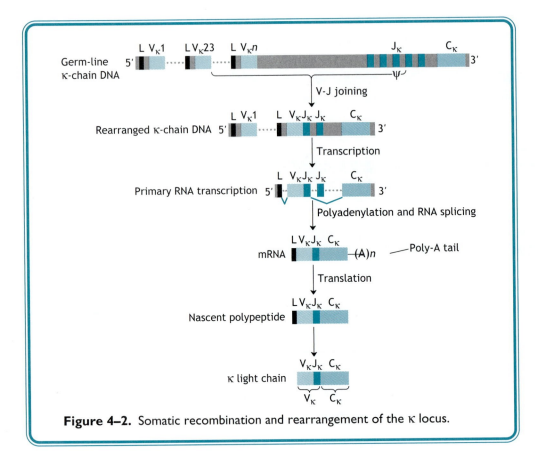

Figure 4–2. Somatic recombination and rearrangement of the κ locus.

RAG DEFICIENCY

CLINICAL CORRELATION

- *Mutations in the Rag1 or Rag2 genes dramatically alter lymphocyte differentiation and cause **severe combined immune deficiency (SCID)**.*
- *SCID is characterized by $T^-B^-NK^+$ lymphopenia, because neither immature B cells nor thymocytes survive differentiation if they cannot successfully express their antigen receptor genes.*
- *SCID is a pediatric emergency due to the rapid onset of fatal opportunistic infections by intracellular pathogens (primarily viral and fungal) early in postnatal life.*
- *Hematopoietic stem cell transplantation in the early neonatal period is a highly successful treatment for SCID.*

4. Sequences within the noncoding introns, called **recombination signal sequences**, determine which gene segments can be juxtaposed by recombination.
5. Additional enzymes catalyze the repair of these double-stranded DNA breaks.
6. The joining of a V segment to a J segment (**V–J joining**) results in the looping out and loss of intervening V and J segments.
7. Any J segments not joined to the V segment as well as intervening introns are excised at the RNA processing stage.
8. The same processes occur at the λ locus.

C. Recombination at the κ and λ loci occurs primarily in the bone marrow independent of any exposure to foreign antigen.

D. Once rearranged, the κ locus can be transcribed into a primary RNA transcript (Figure 4–2).
    1. Rearrangement permits the expression of the κ locus by positioning promoters and enhancers close to one another and the transcriptional start site.
    2. Transcription ends at a stop codon that follows the rearranged C_κ segment.
    3. Intervening RNA and nonjoined J_κ segments are removed by processing the primary RNA transcript.
    4. A messenger RNA (mRNA) is produced by splicing and is then polyadenylated and translated into a κ chain polypeptide.

E. The same process permits the expression of a rearranged λ locus.

CHROMOSOMAL TRANSLOCATIONS TO IG LOCI

• *Many malignant lymphoid cells, including Burkitt s lymphoma and multiple myeloma, show chromosomal translocations that involve the Ig loci.*

• *The high level of genetic recombination that occurs at Ig loci during lymphocyte development makes them particularly susceptible to these genetic abnormalities.*

• *Particularly frequent are translocations that include oncogenes, such as c-myc.*

• *Translocating genes for growth factors, various growth factor receptors, antiapoptosis genes (eg, bcl-2), and transcription factors to the transcriptionally active Ig loci can promote uncontrolled cell proliferation.*

F. The process of gene rearrangement at the H chain locus is slightly different (Figure 4–3).
    1. The first rearrangement involves the joining of a D segment with a J segment (**D–J joining**).
    2. Following D–J joining, the V region is joined to the D–J segment by a second recombination.
    3. Intervening D, J, and V regions are deleted during these recombinations.
    4. H locus rearrangement occurs only in pre-B cells (Chapter 9).
    5. Transcription yields a primary RNA transcript consisting of joined $V_H D_H J_H C_\mu C_\delta$ segments.
        a. Transcription is initiated by promoters upstream of the joined V_H segment.
        b. The first downstream stop codon for transcription is found downstream of the C_δ segment.
            (1) There is no stop codon following the C_μ segment.
            (2) Primary transcripts from the rearranged H locus have the capacity to encode complete μ and δ polypeptide chains.
            (3) The same $V_H D_H J_H$-encoding region is shared by the μ and δ mRNA (see below).
    6. A primary RNA transcript is synthesized, processed, polyadenylated, and translated into an Ig H chain.
    7. Assembly of H and L polypeptide chains occurs in the rough endoplasmic reticulum.
    8. Glycosylation and packaging for secretion occur within the Golgi.

G. The random process of recombination that occurs within each B cell adds to the diversity of the entire B cell pool.

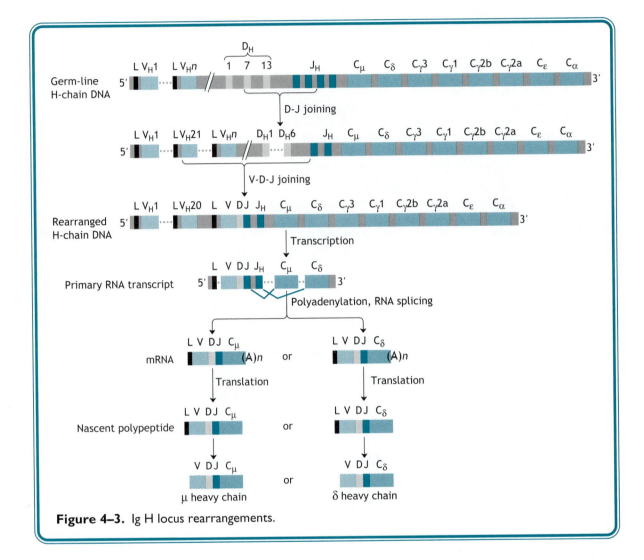

Figure 4–3. Ig H locus rearrangements.

H. A relatively small pool consisting of several hundred V, D, and J segments recombines to generate a very large potential pool ($> 10^{10}$) of V region-encoding genes (Table 4–1).

I. **Allelic exclusion** ensures that a single B cell expresses no more than one BCR.
   1. Diploid species have an opportunity to express both alleles at a given locus.
   2. Successful rearrangements at one allele signal inhibition of rearrangements at the homologous allele.
      a. If rearrangement at the first H-chain locus is nonproductive, rearrangement is attempted at the second H locus.
      b. If the first allele rearranges successfully, rearrangement at the second allele is inhibited.
      c. If both alleles fail to productively rearrange, the cell may undergo apoptosis.

Table 4–1. Various mechanisms contribute to the diversity in Ig molecules.

Mechanism	κ	λ	H
A pool of V, D, and J segments	40 V segments 5 J segments	30 V segments 4 J segments	50 V segments 27 D segments 6 J segments
Combinations of VDJ joining	$40 \times 5 = 200$	$30 \times 4 = 120$	$51 \times 27 \times 6 = 8262$
Imprecise joining	Significant amplification	Significant amplification	Significant amplification
Nucleotide addition or deletion	Significant amplification	Significant amplification	Significant amplification
Combinations of H + L polypeptides[a]	(200	+ 120)	$\times 8262 = 2.64 \times 10^6$
BCR editing[b]	+	+	+
Somatic hypermutation[b]	+	+	+

[a]This estimate of the potential Ig repertoire does not include the amplification derived from imprecise joining and nucleotide additions or deletions.
[b]The effects of these processes are difficult to estimate, can depend upon exposure to antigen, and affect both L and H chain gene expression (Chapter 9). BCR, B cell receptor.

   d. Successful rearrangement of either κ allele inhibits rearrangements at both of the λ loci.
   e. Failing to rearrange both κ alleles signals rearrangement at the λ locus.

IV. Antibody diversity has a genetic basis.

   A. The **immune repertoire** of an individual is the sum of his or her Ig and TCR V regions.
   B. Several mechanisms contribute to the generation of the **potential Ig repertoire** (Table 4–1).
     1. Hundreds of V, D, and J segments are present in the germ line that can combine to code for Ig V regions.
     2. **Combinatorial association** of these segments in a random fashion adds diversity.
     3. **Imprecise joining (joining flexibility)** can generate several sequence variations spanning the recombined region.
     4. **Nucleotide addition or deletion** can occur at joining sites during recombination.
        a. Nucleotides are added by the enzyme **terminal deoxynucleotidyltransferase (TdT)** to generate **junctional diversity.**

b. Because the HV3 region of Ig polypeptides is encoded by the sites of V(D)J joining, junctional diversity is greatest within this hypervariable region (Figure 4–3).

     5. Combinatorial pairing of H and L polypeptide chains further expands the potential repertoire of Ig molecules.

     6. Somatic hypermutation of V region sequences and **BCR editing** (Chapter 9) add to the diversity of mature B cell specificities.

  C. The **utilized repertoire** of an individual can be different from the potential repertoire of the species.

     1. Many recombinations are nonproductive and signal either cell death or a second recombination event.

     2. Some V regions show specificity for self antigens resulting in the deletion of the clone expressing those antigen receptors.

     3. Some H and L polypeptide chains do not pair to form functional antigen receptors.

     4. At any one time the host may not possess sufficient numbers of B cells to accommodate expression of all potential BCR of the species.

     5. Any expansion in a clone of effector or memory B cells can reduce the size of the available repertoire by limiting the space for newly emerging naive B cells with novel specificities.

     6. The generation of memory B cells can increase the repertoire by signaling somatic hypermutation of V regions (Chapter 9).

V. A single B cell can express BCRs of different Ig classes.

  A. A mature naive B cell in the periphery expresses both μ- and δ-containing membrane BCRs.

     1. The primary RNA transcribed from a rearranged H locus gene contains exons for both μ and δ constant regions (Figure 4–4).

         a. Differential processing of the RNA produces mRNAs that code for either μ or δ H chains.

         b. The VDJ sequences of the two mRNA species are the same.

     2. These two BCRs differ from one another only in their C_H domains.

         a. The V regions and L chains of the two BCRs are identical.

         b. The idiotypes and specificities of the two BCRs are identical.

     3. At different stages in the differentiation of B cells (Chapter 9), RNA processing and translation determine whether membrane IgM, membrane IgD, or both are expressed by the cell.

BICLONAL MYELOMA

- *Very rarely patients with multiple myeloma will synthesize two different M components in their plasma.*
- *These monoclonal Igs belong to different Ig classes (eg, IgM and IgG) but typically have identical V region sequences.*
- *Antiidiotype antibodies specific for the combining site of one M protein react with the combining site of the second M protein.*
- *The disease process of myeloma is thought to begin at the pre-B or immature B cell stage, at which time V(D)J sequences are being established by recombination.*
- *Commitment to the H chain class occurs later, during which these rare multiple isotypic neoplasias arise.*

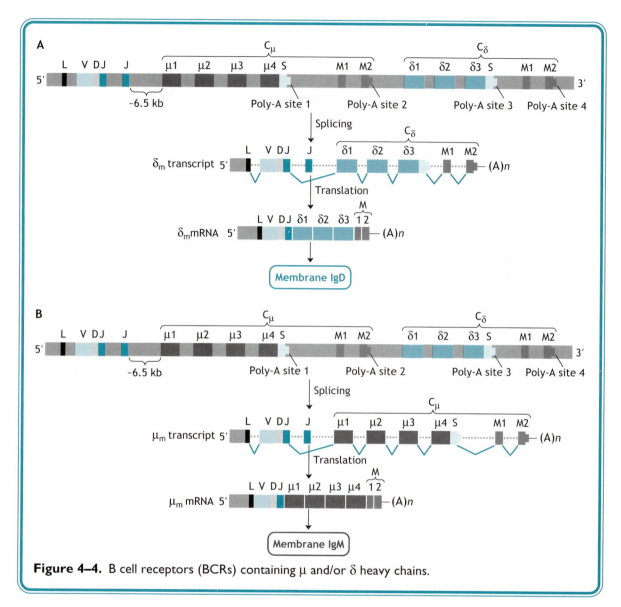

Figure 4–4. B cell receptors (BCRs) containing μ and/or δ heavy chains.

B. Normal B cells maintain their specificity as they undergo Ig class switching following antigen stimulation.

1. **Class (or isotype) switching** refers to a change from the expression of IgM and IgD to the expression of one of the other isotypes (ie, IgG).

   a. Class switching involves a change in the C_H region of the heavy polypeptide chain of the Ig molecule.

   b. During class switching, the L chain remains the same.

   c. The V_H and V_L regions of the Ig, which determine specificity, remain the same during class switching.

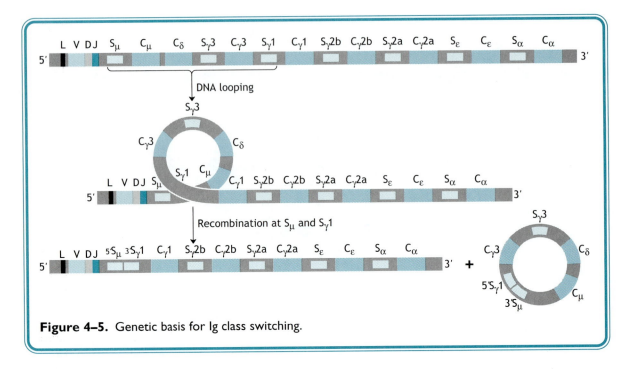

Figure 4–5. Genetic basis for Ig class switching.

2. At the DNA level, Ig class switching involves a change in the order of the C_H segments (Figure 4–5).
a. DNA between the rearranged VDJ segment and the new C_H segment is looped out by recombination.
b. Class switching is irreversible, because the intervening DNA is excised and discarded.
c. Isotype switching always involves a new *downstream* ($3'$) C_H gene segment.
d. A switch from IgM and IgD to IgG expression, for example, can be followed by a second switch to another isotype (eg, IgE).

C. Membrane Ig H chains differ from the secreted form of the same polypeptide only in the presence of membrane-spanning domains at their carboxy-termini (Figure 4–4).
1. A single primary RNA transcript is differentially processed to yield two different mRNAs that encode for either membrane or secreted heavy chains.
2. All of the Ig isotypes have membrane and secreted forms.
3. The membrane antigen receptor (BCR) and secreted antibody molecules of a clone of B cells have the same idiotype and specificity.

VI. Defining the genetic basis for Ig diversity and expression explains much of the unique behavior of B cells (Table 4–2).

A. B cells express antigen receptors that are membrane-bound forms of secreted antibody molecules.

B. Allelic exclusion ensures that the BCR expressed by a B cell is monospecific.

Table 4–2. Molecular correlates of the clonal selection theory.

Prediction	Molecular Explanation
Lymphocytes are precommitted in their antigen specificity.	Gene rearrangement occurs in each lymphocyte during its differentiation in the bone marrow and thymus.
A single cell expresses receptors with a uniform antigen specificity.	Rearrangements that lead to BCR[a] or TCR[a] expression are followed by the inhibition of further Ig or TCR locus rearrangements (allelic exclusion).
All antigen receptors on a cell are uniform and identical.	Each antigen receptor variant on a cell uses the same rearranged V region segments.
Daughter cells retain the antigen specificity of the parental cell.	Once expressed, V region genes are relatively stable in lymphocytes.
The antigen receptor of a cell has a specificity identical to the antibody the cell produces.	The same V regions are used to encode for membrane and secreted Ig molecules.

[a]BCR, B cell receptor; TCR, T cell receptor.

C. The antigenic specificity of a B cell is maintained throughout its life span despite clonal expansion, memory cell production, antibody secretion, and isotype switching.

D. T cells utilize many of the same mechanisms to express an even more diverse set of antigen receptors.

CLINICAL PROBLEMS

Mary is a 3-year-old patient who presents with a fever, labored breathing, and shortness of breath. Her history includes recurrent bacterial infections (sinusitis and otitis media) since 1 year of age. She has been prescribed oral antibiotics as often as six times per year. After each course of treatment, the infections subside, but a recurrence of symptoms often follows within several weeks. Laboratory tests indicate a mild neutropenia, but no other hematological abnormalities. Her serum IgG and IgA levels are far below those of age-matched controls, whereas her serum IgM levels are significantly elevated. When immunized with tetanus toxoid, a vaccine she has received before, she makes no detectable IgG antibody response.

1. Which of the following is the most likely cellular or molecular defect in this patient?

    A. Failure of her B cells to undergo Ig class switching

    B. A block in all B cell differentiation

    C. Rag1 deficiency

    D. Toll-like receptor deficiency

    E. DiGeorge syndrome

A 2-year-old patient presents with a history of infections that suggests an immune defect, and the clinical laboratory reports serum IgG levels one-third that of age-matched controls. The child is ABO blood type A.

2. Which of the following findings would be more consistent with a diagnosis of H locus deletion affecting only C_γ segments than a complete absence of B cells?

    A. Decreased IgM levels in her serum

    B. The absence of follicles in her splenic white pulp

    C. The absence of Ig in her saliva

    D. The presence of B cells in the follicles of her lymph nodes

    E. The lack of isohemagglutinins in her serum

You have isolated a population of plasma cells from a patient who was recently immunized with a protein vaccine. Her cells secrete IgG in vitro, but lack any membrane IgG.

3. Which of the following accounts for this finding?

    A. DNA rearrangement following antigen stimulation deletes BCR-encoding gene segments.

    B. The Ig H chain locus does not code for a membrane form of γ chains.

    C. Differential RNA processing favors the synthesis of a secreted form of γ heavy chains.

    D. Plasma cells that secrete IgG express IgA on their surface.

    E. Only surface L chains are expressed by B cells.

You have a patient with an $IgG_1\kappa$ myeloma. Analysis of DNA from the myeloma cells indicates that the H and κ alleles that he inherited from his father (paternal) have been rearranged.

4. Which of the following loci could still be in the germ line configuration in these cells?

    A. Maternal κ allele

    B. Maternal λ allele

    C. Paternal λ allele

    D. Maternal H allele

    E. All of the above loci could be in the germ line configuration.

You have a patient with multiple myeloma and examine a preparation of cellular mRNA from the myeloma cells by Northern blotting. The probe you use detects a $V_H D_H J_H$ sequence that is unique to this particular myeloma cell. The results of this experiment indicate that the myeloma cells have four mRNA species of different sizes, each containing the target sequence.

5. Which one of the following lists of Ig polypeptides is probably encoded by these four mRNAs?

   A. μ, δ, γ, and α H chains

   B. κ, λ, μ, and δ chains

   C. Membrane μ, membrane δ, secreted μ, and secreted δ H chains

   D. Secreted μ, δ, κ, and λ chains

   E. Secreted μ, δ, α, and ε H chains

ANSWERS

1. The correct answer is A. Mary produces IgM, which rules out an absence of B cells or a Rag deficiency. The latter would cause a complete absence of both T and B cells, which would have resulted in the onset of viral and fungal infections shortly after birth. Mary's history of infections, serum IgG and IgA levels, and diminished antibody response suggest that she lacks the ability to class switch from IgM production to the more "mature" isotypes (IgG and IgA).

2. The correct answer is D. With γ chain gene deletions, mature B cells are still produced and can be found in the periphery. They simply fail to synthesize IgG antibodies after antigen stimulation. With a complete absence of B cells, follicles in the lymph nodes and spleen fail to develop.

3. The correct answer is C. Whereas mature B lymphocytes express membrane BCR molecules, plasma cells do not normally express membrane Ig. This decision in the B cell lineage to express membrane Ig, secreted Ig, or both is made at the level of RNA processing.

4. The correct answer is E. The H locus rearranges first, followed by either the κ or λ locus. If successful rearrangements had first been undertaken at the paternal H and κ alleles, then the maternal H and κ alleles would remain in the germ line arrangement. Because the κ locus was successfully rearranged in this cell, both λ alleles could have been suppressed and could have remained in the germ line configuration.

5. The correct answer is C. Because the probe detects only mRNAs with VDJ sequences of H chains, light chain mRNA should not be detected. Messenger RNA for μ and δ chains could be expressed by one myeloma cell by differential splicing, and these mRNA would differ only in their C_H regions. μ and δ H chains have different molecular masses, and their membrane forms, which are expressed by a portion of the myeloma cells, are longer than their secreted forms.

CHAPTER 5
ANTIGEN RECOGNITION BY ANTIBODY

I. Interactions between antibodies and antigens are specific, reversible, and reach a state of equilibrium defined by the following equation:

$$Ab + Ag \leftrightarrows AbAg$$

A. The molecular forces that contribute to the strength of antibody–antigen (Ab–Ag) binding include ionic bonding, hydrophobic interactions, hydrogen bonding, and van der Waals interactions.

1. Affinity is a measure of the strength of binding between an antibody and a monovalent antigen.

   a. Antibody affinities are reflected in **dissociation constants** (K_d) and typically range from 10^{-6} to 10^{-11} M.

   b. The average affinity of an antiserum generally increases with repeated immunizations, a phenomenon referred to as **affinity maturation** (Chapter 9).

   c. As a general rule, immunoglobulin (Ig) G antibodies have higher affinities than IgM antibodies.

2. Antibody avidity refers to the aggregate strength of Ab–Ag binding when multiple antibody-combining sites of an antibody molecule interact with more than one determinant of a multivalent antigen.

   a. High avidity reactions are common with natural antigens that contain multiple copies of the same antigenic determinant (eg, polysaccharides).

   b. Because of their pentameric structure, IgM antibodies generally have a higher avidity than IgG antibodies.

B. The **specificity** of Ab–Ag reactions is similar to the specificity that enzymes show for their substrates.

1. Antibodies can distinguish between sterioisomeric forms of chemical groups.

2. Cross-reactivity is the tendency of an antibody to react with more than one antigen.

   a. Cross-reactive antigens (eg, bovine and equine serum albumin) share the same or similar antigenic determinants.

   b. In general, **polyclonal antisera** are more cross-reactive than **monoclonal antibodies**.

   c. B cell and T cell receptors (BCR and TCR) can also show cross-reactivity (Chapter 6).

CROSS-REACTIVITY AND CROSS-PROTECTION

- *Immunity induced by vaccination, infection, or environmental exposure to antigens can lead to either beneficial or deleterious immunological cross-reactions (Table 5–1).*
- *Edward Jenner developed an effective means of eliciting cross-protective immunity to the variola (smallpox) virus by immunizing individuals with vaccinia virus, which causes cowpox.*
- *The nonpathogenic mycobacterium bacille Calmette-Guérin (BCG) induces in vaccinees cross-protective immunity against the causative agent of tuberculosis, Mycobacterium tuberculosis.*
- *Allergic responses to cross-reactive determinants on birch pollen can lead to food allergies to apples, plums, and hazelnuts.*

    C. When antibodies bind to their respective antigens, neither is covalently modified, although both can undergo important conformational changes.

      1. Some cell surface **Fcγ receptors** bind IgG Fc regions only after they have bound antigen.

        a. These Fcγ receptors are generally of low affinity (K_d = 10^{-6}–10^{-7} M) and mediate opsonization by phagocytic cells.

        b. High affinity Fcγ and Fcε receptors (K_d = 10^{-8}–10^{-10} M) can bind monomeric IgG and IgE, respectively, in the absence of antigen.

        c. High-affinity Fc receptors mediate placental transfer of monomeric IgG.

      2. The activation of **complement** by IgG and IgM antibodies requires antigen binding that reveals cryptic complement-binding sites within the C_H2 domains (Chapter 8).

      3. Membrane Igs that serve as antigen receptors on B cells undergo conformational changes when their antigens are bound.

        a. This permits protein–protein interactions between the C-terminal domains of membrane H chains and two other members of the receptor complex, Igα and Igβ.

        b. BCR–Igα–Igβ interactions initiate transmembrane signaling in B cells (Chapter 9).

Table 5–1. Clinically important immunological crossreactions.

Antibody Specificity	Cross-reactive Antigens	Effect
Microbial carbohydrates	ABO erythrocyte antigens	Mediate transfusion reactions
Steptococcal M protein	Cardiac antigens	Rheumatic fever
Beef heart cardiolipin	Human cardiolipin	False positive tests for syphilis
House dust mite allergens	Shrimp	Food allergies
Timothy grass allergens	June grass allergens	Seasonal allergies
Methyldopa	Rh antigens	Autoimmune hemolytic anemia

D. A complex formed between an antibody and its antigen is often referred to as an **immune complex**.

1. Both circulating and tissue-bound immune complexes have proinflammatory effects (Chapter 13).

2. Circulating soluble immune complexes typically form in antigen excess and deposit in the skin, blood vessel walls, joint spaces, and basement membranes of renal glomeruli.

3. A number of important laboratory tests can detect immune complexes in body fluids or tissues and aid in diagnosing **immune complex diseases** (Chapters 13 and 16).

II. The measurement of Ab–Ag reactions is the basis for many clinical diagnostic tests in immunology and microbiology (Table 5–2).

A. Serology refers to techniques that measure the reactivity of serum antibodies with their antigens.

Table 5–2. Selected applications of immunoassays in the clinical laboratory.[a]

Measurement	Assay	Specific Examples
Ig concentration	Nephelometry	Serum IgG, IgM, IgA, and IgE
Monoclonal gammopathy	Immunoelectrophoresis Immunofixation	M component
Complement Individual components Total hemolytic activity	ELISA Complement fixation test	C1, C2, C3, C4 CH_{50}
Antibodies to infectious agents HIV *Streptococcus* *Treponema pallidum*	ELISA, Western blot Agglutination Agglutination	Anti-gp24, gp41, gp120, gp160 Anticapsular polysaccharide VDRL test for syphilis
Autoimmunity Anti-Ig antibody	Passive hemagglutination	Rheumatoid factor
Antinuclear antibodies	Immunofluorescence	ANA, anti-dsDNA
Cell surface markers Normal lymphocytes Tumor cells	Flow cytometry Flow cytometry	CD4, CD8, CD19 CD10 on leukemia cells

[a]Ig, immunoglobulin; ELISA, enzyme-linked immunosorbent assay; HIV, human immunodeficiency virus; VDRL, Venereal Disease Research Laboratory; ANA, antinuclear antibody; dsDNA, double-stranded DNA.

B. The relative concentration of an antibody is often expressed as a **titer**, which is the reciprocal of the greatest dilution of the antiserum that shows a reaction with its antigen.

C. Particulate antigens agglutinate when combined with their antibodies.

1. Hemagglutination occurs when antibodies to erythrocyte surface antigens cause aggregation of cells bearing the respective antigen.

a. In **blood typing**, agglutinating antibodies of known specificities (eg, anti-RhD) are used to determine the antigenic phenotypes of prospective donors and recipients.

b. In the **major cross-match**, cells from the donor are mixed with serum from the recipient as a means of detecting preformed recipient antidonor antibodies.

2. The **Coombs test** (Chapter 16), a specialized hemagglutination test, detects antibodies on erythrocytes or platelets.

a. In the Coombs test, the patient's cells are mixed with the **"Coombs reagent,"** which is an antihuman IgG.

b. IgG antibody-coated erythrocytes or platelets agglutinate in the presence of the Coombs reagent.

c. Agglutination can indicate the presence of antibodies against haptens (eg, drugs) bound to the cell surface or antibodies specific for endogenous erythrocyte antigens (eg, anti-RhD).

RH DISEASE OF THE NEWBORN

• *Rh incompatibility between Rh-negative mothers and their Rh-positive children can lead to the production of antibodies by the mother that cause hemolytic anemia in the fetus.*

• *First pregnancies are generally not affected, because the initial maternal IgM antibodies do not cross the placenta.*

• *Subsequent pregnancies are at risk due to isotype switching to IgG in the mother.*

• *A definitive diagnosis of Rh disease in an affected newborn can be made, in part, with the Coombs test, which detects IgG on the surface of the neonate's erythrocytes.*

3. The species or strain of a bacterium can be determined by serological agglutination tests.

a. Serological typing provides a more rapid identification of a bacterial species or group (eg, group A *Streptococcus* or *Salmonella* serogroups) than does culturing the specimen.

b. Agglutination assays can also reveal serotypes associated with specific diseases (eg, *Escherichia coli* serotype O157:H7 and hemorrhagic colitis).

D. Soluble antigens present at high concentrations form visible precipitates when combined with their antibodies.

1. Immunoprecipitation techniques are relatively insensitive and require microgram per milliliter to milligram per milliliter concentrations of antigen.

2. Large insoluble Ab–Ag precipitates can be detected by light scatter using an instrument known as a **nephelometer**.

3. The amount of immune precipitate that forms is a function of the Ab:Ag ratio (Figure 5–1).

a. At an optimum ratio, called **equivalence**, the maximum amount of precipitate is observed and neither free Ab nor free Ag is found in solution.

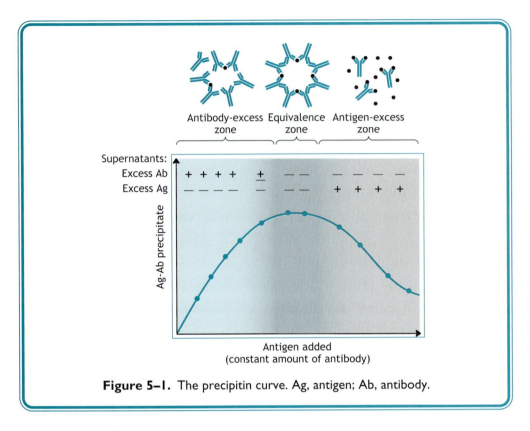

Figure 5–1. The precipitin curve. Ag, antigen; Ab, antibody.

    b. In the range of **Ag excess**, small soluble Ab_1Ag_2 complexes are formed.

    c. Large complexes are typically cleared by phagocytic cells, whereas smaller soluble complexes can cause **immune complex disease**.

4. Precipitated Ab–Ag complexes can also be visualized in agar gels.

    a. In **agar gel immunodiffusion**, solutions of Ab and Ag diffuse toward one another resulting in the formation of a visible precipitate at the diffusion interface (Figure 5–2).

        (1) A pattern of **identity** indicates that two antigens are identical with respect to the determinant(s) recognized by the antiserum.

        (2) A pattern of **partial identity** occurs when two antigens share some, but not all, of their antigenic determinants.

        (3) A pattern of **nonidentity** forms when two antigens have unique determinants not found in the other.

    b. **Immunofixation**, which combines the technique of electrophoresis with immunoprecipitation, is used to analyze antigens in complex biological samples, such as serum (Figure 5–3).

        (1) Test samples are first electrophoresed in an agar gel.

        (2) The electrophoresed proteins are then detected with specific antibodies that precipitate the antigen.

        (3) These insoluble immune precipitates are stained with a protein stain.

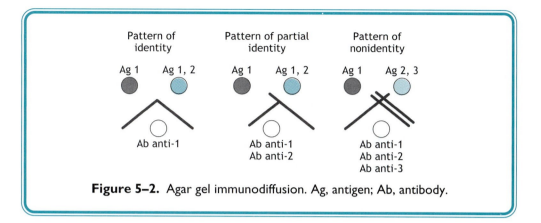

Figure 5–2. Agar gel immunodiffusion. Ag, antigen; Ab, antibody.

POLYCLONAL AND MONOCLONAL GAMMOPATHIES

- *Hypergammaglobulinemia* can occur following repeated immunization, infection, or abnormal B cell differentiation, including neoplasia.
- A **polyclonal gammopathy** generally signals infection, whereas a **monoclonal gammopathy** indicates a benign or malignant condition affecting a single clone of B cells.
- Benign **monoclonal gammopathy of undetermined significance (MGUS)** is common in the elderly, occurring at a frequency of approximately 3% in persons over 70 years of age.
- Because many monoclonal conditions are malignant, it is important to determine whether a hypergammaglobulinemia is monoclonal.
- Immunofixation is used to ascertain whether the elevated γ-globulins have a single H chain class and L chain type, which means they are likely monoclonal.

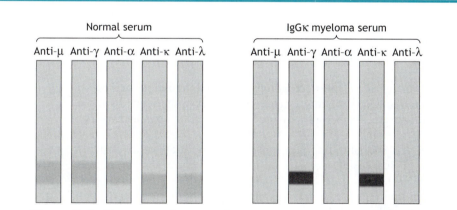

Figure 5–3. Detection of a monoclonal gammopathy by immunofixation.

E. Sensitive immunoassays are required to detect antigens that exist at low concentrations (picogram per milliliter to nanogram per milliliter) in clinical samples.

    1. Radioimmunoassays use radiolabeled antigens or antibodies.

        a. The competitive radioimmunoassay measures the ability of a test sample (eg, patient serum) to compete with a radiolabeled antigen for binding to an immobilized antibody.

        b. Immunoassays of this type require that dilutions of purified antigen be included as standards.

        c. The **radioallergosorbant test** is a radioimmunoassay that measures the concentration of serum IgE antibody to a known allergen (Chapter 13).

    2. Enzyme-linked immunosorbent assays (EIA or ELISA) use enzyme-conjugated antibodies (E-Ab) to detect antigens.

        a. The E-Ab–Ag complexes are detected by their ability to convert a chromogenic substrate into a colored product.

        b. Like radioimmunoassay (RIA), the ELISA can be used to measure antigen or antibody concentrations and shows sensitivity for antigens in solution in the picogram per milliliter range.

        c. Many **home pregnancy tests** use ELISA technology to detect human chorionic gonadotropin in the urine.

    3. Immunoblotting (Western blotting) uses either radiolabeled or enzyme-conjugated antibodies to detect antigens within a complex sample, such as serum or a tissue extract.

        a. The sample is first electrophoresed in a polyacrylamide gel under conditions that separate antigens according to their molecular weights.

        b. Separated proteins are then transferred from the gel to a membrane.

        c. The membrane is treated with an E-Ab.

        d. E-Ab–Ag complexes are detected by incubating the membrane with a chromogenic substrate, which forms an insoluble colored precipitate on the complex.

        e. Western blots are often used to confirm initial screening tests, such as an ELISA.

F. Immunofluorescence assays use fluorescenated antibodies to detect tissue- or cell-bound antigens.

    1. Because of their specificity, the most popular antibodies for this purpose are monoclonal antibodies.

    2. The availability of multiple fluorochromes (dyes) enables polychromatic analysis of more than one antigen at a time.

    3. Specialized equipment (eg, a fluorescence or confocal microscope or flow cytometer) is required to detect the fluorescence emitted from the stained sample.

    4. Tissue immunofluorescence is routinely used to enumerate certain markers in tissue sections (eg, tumors).

    5. Flow cytometry is a specialized application of immunofluorescence in which individual cells in suspension are analyzed for the expression of a given marker(s)(Figure 5–4).

        a. The cell suspension (eg, blood) is first treated with the fluorescenated antibody to label the cell subset of interest.

        b. The labeled cell suspension is then sprayed across the path of a laser to excite the fluorochrome.

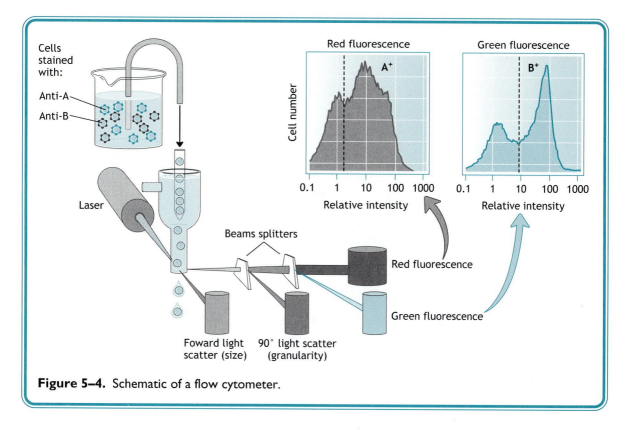

Figure 5–4. Schematic of a flow cytometer.

c. Individual cells are scored for their intensity of fluorescence emission.
d. Flow cytometry is the preferred technique for enumerating CD markers on human cells (Appendix I).
e. **Polychromatic flow cytometry** simultaneously detects multiple markers on a single cell (Figure 5–5).
f. Individual cells expressing these markers can be physically purified by a modification of flow cytometry called **fluorescence-activated cell sorting (FACS)**.

PHENOTYPING LYMPHOMAS AND LEUKEMIAS BY FLOW CYTOMETRY

• *An important application of flow cytometry is the phenotyping of hematological malignancies using monoclonal antibodies to various CD markers.*

• *This approach can establish the number of different cell populations present in a sample, their lineage, and their stage of differentiation.*

• *For example, a typical B cell chronic lymphocytic leukemia (B cell-CLL) expresses membrane Ig, CD5, CD19, CD20, and CD22.*

• *By comparison, a plasmacytoma typically does not express membrane Ig, CD19, CD20, or CD22, but contains intracytoplasmic Ig.*

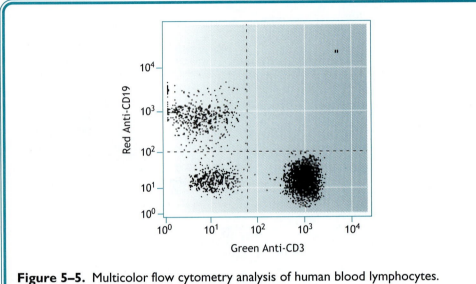

Figure 5–5. Multicolor flow cytometry analysis of human blood lymphocytes.

CLINICAL PROBLEMS

A 1-year-old child with a history of chronic sinusitis, otitis media, and pneumonia is suspected of having a primary immune deficiency. He has benefited from antibiotics and intravenous immunoglobulins and shows a very low concentration of serum IgG and no IgM. Analysis of the patient's lymph node cells by flow cytometry shows normal numbers of CD3+ lymphocytes, but an absence of cells expressing membrane IgM.

1. Which of the following diagnoses is most consistent with the data presented for this patient?

   A. Severe combined immune deficiency (SCID)

   B. X-linked agammaglobulinemia (XLA)

   C. Selective IgG deficiency

   D. Light chain disease

   E. B cell chronic lymphocytic leukemia

You decide to determine whether the patient in question 1 can mount a secondary antibody response to tetanus toxoid. Ten days after immunizing with the toxoid, you measure the titer of serum antibodies to the foreign protein.

2. Which of the following laboratory tests would be most appropriate for measuring this response?

   A. Flow cytometry

   B. ELISA

   C. Immunofluorescence

D. Immunoblotting (Western blotting)

E. Immunodiffusion in gels

You have a patient with recurrent infections and decide to examine a biopsy of her lymph node for potential structural abnormalities. Immunohistological staining reveals very few cells in the diffuse cortex that stain with a peroxidase-conjugated antibody to CD3 followed by a chromogenic peroxidase substrate. Unstained cells are present in the superficial cortex of the lymph node.

3. Which of the following diseases is consistent with this finding?

A. Toll-like receptor deficiency

B. Severe combined immunodeficiency (SCID)

C. Chronic granulomatous disease

D. DiGeorge syndrome

E. Multiple myeloma

A 32-year-old patient presents with lymphopenia, but no other hematological abnormalities. He has mucocutaneous candidiasis, a yeast infection of the mucous membranes, and is seronegative for HIV-1 by ELISA.

4. Which of the following flow cytometry findings with blood lymphocytes [peripheral blood mononuclear cells (PMBCs)] would nonetheless still support a diagnosis of HIV infection in this patient?

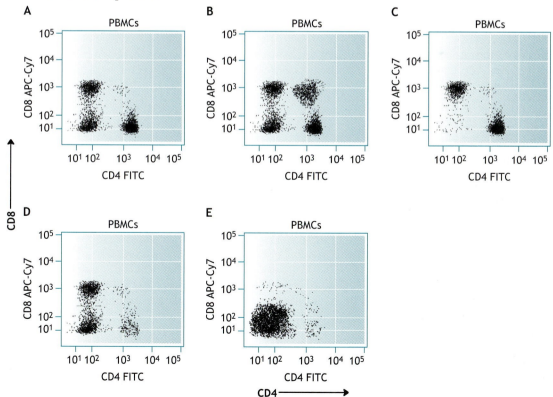

A. Panel A

B. Panel B

C. Panel C

D. Panel D

E. Panel E

A patient with multiple myeloma shows proteinuria, and you wish to characterize the urinary protein. Using immunodiffusion, you react a rabbit antiserum specific for human IgG with the patient's serum and her urine.

5. Which of the patterns shown below would suggest that the urinary protein is an Ig L chain?

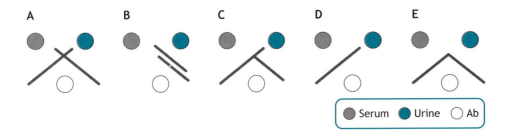

A. Pattern A

B. Pattern B

C. Pattern C

D. Pattern D

E. Pattern E

ANSWERS

1. The correct answer is B. The history and flow cytometry data are consistent with an antibody deficiency that results from the absence of peripheral B cells. Although SCID would also show aberrant B cell differentiation, T cells would be absent in this disease as well.

2. The correct answer is B. Among the choices, only ELISA is a quantitative assay. Immunoblotting is not quantitative, and immunodiffusion requires high concentrations of antibody and antigen to visualize immune precipitates.

3. The correct answer is D. DiGeorge syndrome (thymic dysplasia) results in a selective deficiency of T cells and an acellular appearance in T cell-dependent areas of the lymph nodes.

4. The correct answer is D. There is a selective depletion of CD4⁺ T cells in patients with HIV infections. For a comparison with the normal pattern, see panel A. The pattern in panel B is not typical for blood because it contains double-positive cells, which are normally seen only in the thymus.

5. The correct answer is C. The excess urinary proteins in myeloma are generally Ig L chains (Bence–Jones proteins), which would show a cross-reaction with the patient's serum monoclonal Ig (M component). Because the serum Ig would contain antigenic determinants on their H chains not found on the urinary L chains, a pattern of partial identity would appear.

CHAPTER 6
T CELL RECOGNITION OF AND RESPONSE TO ANTIGEN

I. The T cell receptor (TCR) for antigen is a complex consisting of an antigen-specific heterodimer (TCR) and four additional peptides of the CD3 family (Figure 2–5).

A. TCR structure is similar to that of the B cell receptor (BCR) (Table 6–1).
1. The α, β, γ, and δ polypeptides are transmembrane proteins with short cytoplasmic domains.
2. TCR peptides have amino acid sequence homology with Ig peptides and belong to the **immunoglobulin gene superfamily**.
3. Each TCR peptide has a V domain and a C domain (eg, $V_\alpha C_\alpha$ in α chains), which are stabilized by intrachain disulfide bonds.
4. The two V domains (eg, $V_\alpha + V_\beta$) form a monovalent ligand-binding site much like an Ig Fab fragment.
5. The membrane-distal face of the TCRαβ and TCRγδ receptors that contact their ligands has a flat conformation, rather than the cleft seen in immunoglobulins (Igs) (Figure 6–1).
6. Of peripheral T cells 95% bear TCRs composed of αβ heterodimers; the remaining T cells bear TCRs composed of γδ heterodimers.
7. **CD3 γ, δ, ε, and ζ** polypeptide chains are transmembrane signaling components of the receptor complex.
8. The TCR is never expressed without CD3 peptides; the complete CD3 complex is never expressed on the cell surface without a TCR heterodimer.

CD3 DEFICIENCY

CLINICAL CORRELATION

- *Rare immune deficiencies affecting the expression of the TCR result from natural mutations in the CD3 γ and ε chains.*
- *These patients present with severe lymphopenia at birth due to an inability of their thymocytes to signal through an early form of the TCR called the **pre-TCR**, which requires CD3 for its expression.*
- *Without a functional pre-TCR, immature thymocytes do not develop properly and cellular immunity is impaired (Chapter 10).*
- *Opportunistic viral and fungal infections occur early in life and require aggressive treatment.*

B. The expression of TCR genes requires their rearrangement by recombination during cell differentiation in the thymus (Figure 6–2).

64

Table 6–1. Distinguishing features of the BCR and TCR.[a]

Feature	BCR	TCR
Antigen-specific component	Membrane Ig	$\alpha\beta$ or $\gamma\delta$ heterodimer
Receptor valence	Bivalent	Monovalent
Signaling peptides	Igα, Igβ	CD3 γ, δ, ϵ, ζ
Ligand	Native epitopes of proteins, carbohydrates, lipids, nucleic acids	Processed peptides plus MHC or glycolipids plus CD1
Isotype switching	Yes	No

[a]BCR, B cell receptor; TCR, T cell receptor; Ig, immunoglobulin; MHC, major histocompatibility complex.

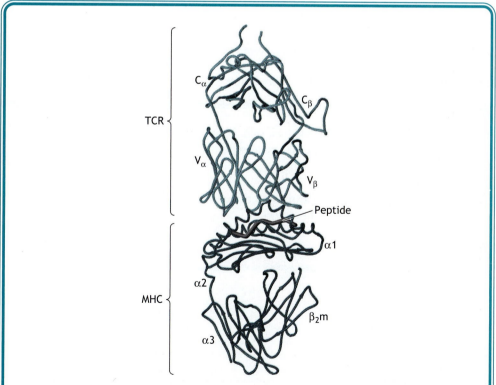

Figure 6–1. Model of a typical T cell receptor (TCR) showing the structure of the ligand-binding surface. MHC, major histocompatibility complex. (Adapted, with permission, from Garcia KC: An $\alpha\beta$T cell receptor structure at 2.5 A and its Orientation in the TCR-MHC complex. Science 1996;274:209.)

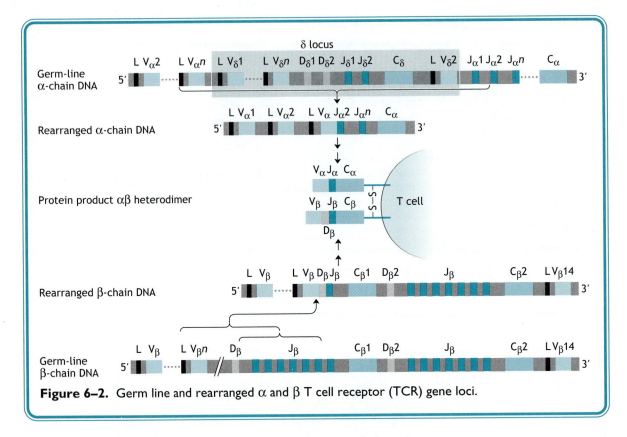

Figure 6–2. Germ line and rearranged α and β T cell receptor (TCR) gene loci.

1. The TCR genes are found at three genetic loci, α/δ, β, and γ.
2. Variable (V), joining (J), and constant (C) gene segments are found at each locus (Table 6–2).
3. Diversity (D) segments are present within the β and δ loci.

C. The diversity of the TCR repertoire arises from genetic mechanisms that are similar to those used to create a diverse set of Ig molecules.

Table 6–2. TCR locus gene segments.[a]

Segment	TCRα	TCRβ	TCRγ	TCRδ
V	50	57	14	3
D	0	2	0	3
J	70	13	5	3
C	1	2	2	1

[a]TCR, T cell receptor.

1. There are several hundred V, D, and J segments that recombine randomly to create a pool of rearranged TCR V genes.
2. Imprecise joining and nucleotide addition add diversity.
3. Combinatorial association between the α and β or the γ and δ chains further expands the repertoire.
4. TCR editing occurs infrequently, and there is no somatic hypermutation of TCR V region sequences as there is for BCR V region genes.

TCR REARRANGEMENTS IN CANCER

- *The molecular diagnosis of human T cell leukemias and lymphomas is greatly aided by showing that they are monoclonal and express a TCR with a uniform V_α or V_β region.*
- *This can be accomplished by molecular techniques, such as the polymerase chain reaction (PCR), that demonstrate the proliferating cells have rearranged a uniform TCR V_α or V_β segment.*
- *This type of molecular approach aids in early diagnosis and monitoring the status of the neoplastic clone during therapy.*

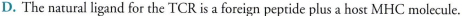

D. The natural ligand for the TCR is a foreign peptide plus a host MHC molecule.
1. The TCR recognizes peptides derived from foreign protein antigens that are bound to a major histocompatibility complex (MHC) molecule and presented by an antigen-presenting cell (APC).
2. The complementarity determining regions (CDRs) of the TCR make contact with amino acid residues of both the peptide and the MHC molecule (Figure 6–1).

E. **Superantigens** produced by microbes can bind the TCR and the MHC outside the peptide-binding site.
1. *Staphylococcus* and *Streptococcus* species produce exotoxins that act as superantigens.
2. Microbial superantigens cross-link TCR V_β regions to MHC class II molecules.
3. Binding of superantigens to the TCR induces polyclonal activation of T cells.

TOXIC SHOCK SYNDROME

- **Toxic shock syndrome (TSS)** *is a systemic disease associated with vaginal or surgical wound infections with the gram-positive bacterium Staphylococcus aureus.*
- *S aureus produces a superantigen, called* **toxic shock syndrome toxin (TSST)**, *which activates CD4$^+$ T cells to produce massive quantities of inflammatory cytokines.*
- *The systemic nature of the inflammatory response manifests as fever, coagulopathies, extreme hypotension, skin rash and exfoliation, and diarrhea.*

F. **Natural killer T (NKT) cells** express an unusual form of the TCR.
1. **Invariant NKT cells (iNKT cells)** express a uniform α chain composed of a single V_α region called $V_\alpha 24$.
2. The β chain of the iNKT cell TCR is created by recombination using only a subset of the V_β gene segments.
3. The known ligands of the iNKT cell TCR are glycolipids that are presented by CD1 molecules, not MHC molecules (Chapter 7).
4. iNKT cells produce cytokines and become cytotoxic when activated through their TCR.

II. Optimum T cell activation by antigen requires TCR stimulation and signals derived from the APC.

A. Compared to antibodies, TCRs bind their ligands with relatively low affinity (K_d 10^4–10^5 M).

B. The binding between a T cell and its APC is strengthened by the T cell **adhesion molecules** LFA-1 and CD2 (Table 6–3).

C. **Coreceptors** on T cells augment the intracellular signal transduction pathways that are initiated by the TCR–CD3 complex.

   1. Many coreceptors promote TCR signaling by phosphorylating **immunotyrosine activation motifs (ITAMs)** of CD3.

   2. T cells that express TCR specific for peptide-MHC *class II* complexes use **CD4** as a signaling coreceptor.

   3. T cells that express TCR specific for peptide-MHC *class I* complexes use **CD8** as a coreceptor.

   4. **CD28** provides important coactivation signaling for T cells.

   5. **CD154** is a ligand for the CD40 coreceptor found on B cells.

D. **Cytokines** provide a second source of costimulatory signals (Chapter 12).

HYPER IGM SYNDROME

CLINICAL CORRELATION

• Children with X-linked **hyper IgM syndrome** show elevated levels of serum IgM, but extremely low concentrations of IgG, IgA, and IgE.

• Their activated T cells lack **CD154**, which results in impaired Th cell function and B cell signaling.

• Impaired Ig class switching in B cells results in elevated IgM antibody levels.

• With the failure to produce opsonizing IgG antibodies, infections with pyogenic (pus-forming) bacteria are common in these patients.

Table 6–3. Adhesion molecules and coreceptors on T cells.[a]

T Cell Coreceptor	Ligand on APC	Cells That Express the Receptor Ligand
LFA-1	ICAM-1	Endothelial cells, many others
CD2	CD58	Many cells
CD4	MHC class II	Dendritic cells, B cells, macrophages
CD8	MHC class I	Nearly all nucleated cells
CD28	B7	Dendritic cells, activated B cells, macrophages
CD154	CD40	Dendritic cells, B cells, macrophages, others

[a]APC, antigen-presenting cell; LFA-1, lymphocyte function-associated antigen 1; ICAM, intercellular adhesion molecule; MHC, major histocompatibility complex.

III. Signaling through the TCR leads to gene transcription.

A. The binding of the TCR to it ligand recruits the CD3 peptides to the αβ chains via charge interactions in their transmembrane domains.

B. **ITAMs** in the cytoplasmic tails of CD3 peptides are sites for the assembly of signaling intermediates, including the kinase **ζ-associated protein-70 kDa (ZAP-70)** (Figure 6–3).

   1. ZAP-70 becomes phosphorylated and, in turn, phosphorylates **phospholipase Cγ (PLCγ)**.

   a. PLCγ hydrolyzes the membrane phospholipid phosphatidylinositol 4,5-biphosphate (PIP_2) producing **diacylglyceride (DAG)** and **inositol 1,4,5-triphosphate (IP_3)**.

   (1) DAG activates **protein kinase C (PKC)**, which activates the **nuclear factor-κB (NFκB)** transcription factor pathway (Figure 6–4).

   (2) IP_3 mobilizes intracellular Ca^{2+}, which activates **calmodulin**.

   (3) Ca^{2+}/calmodulin-dependent enzymes, including the phosphatase **calcineurin**, are activated.

   (4) Calcineurin mediates *de*phosphorylation of the latent transcription factor **nuclear factor of activated T cells (NFAT)**.

   2. ZAP-70 also phosphorylates adapter proteins that lead to the activation of the G protein-mediated Ras/Rac pathways.

   a. **Mitogen-activated protein (MAP) kinases** are then activated.

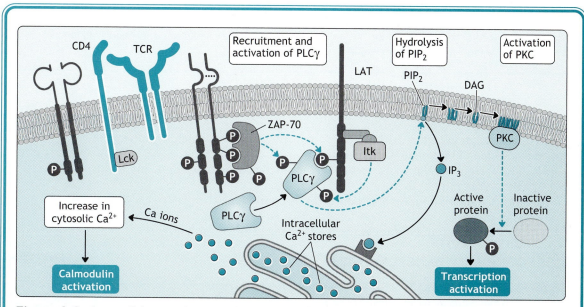

Figure 6–3. Intracellular signaling events accompanying T cell activation. PLC, phospholipase C; PIP_2, phosphatidylinositol 4,5-biphosphate; PKC, protein kinase C; ZAP-70, ζ-associated protein-70 kDa; LAT, linker for activation of T cells; DAG, diacylglyceride; IP_3, inositol 1,4,5-triphosphate.

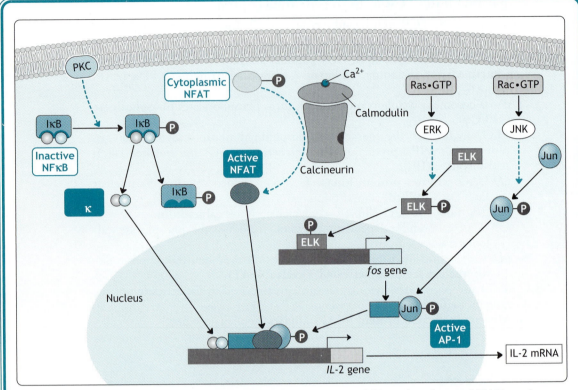

Figure 6–4. Transcription factors that mediate T cell signaling. NF, nuclear factor; NFAT, nuclear factor of activated T cells; GTP, guanosine triphosphate; ERK, extracellular signal-regulated kinase; JNK, Jun N-terminal kinase; IL, interleukin.

    b. The MAP kinases phosphorylate and activate the **AP-1** family of transcription factors (Figure 6–4).

  C. The transcription factors NFκB, NFAT, and AP-1 act coordinately to initiate the transcription of important T cell genes.

    1. NFAT regulates the transcription of the interleukin (IL)-2, IL-4, interferon (IFN)-γ, and tumor necrosis factor (TNF)-α genes.

    2. NFκB transcription factors induce the expression of the IL-2, IFN-γ, and TNF-α genes.

    3. AP-1 activates transcription of the IL-2 and many other cytokine genes.

CYCLOSPORINE AND TRANSPLANTATION

- *Cyclosporine and the related drug FK-506 (Tracolimus) have proven effective in managing allograft rejection episodes that are mediated by activated T cells.*
- *Both drugs inhibit the cellular phosphatase calcineurin and thereby diminish NFAT activation and cytokine gene expression.*
- *The use of these powerful immunosuppressive drugs has allowed clinical transplantation to be performed successfully even when some genetic disparity exists between donor and host (Chapter 17).*

D. Coreceptors augment signaling initiated by the TCR (Figure 6–3).
   1. CD4 and CD8 binding to MHC molecules recruits the kinase **Lck** to the TCR complex.
   2. Lck then phosphorylates the CD3ζ ITAM residues, which promotes ZAP-70 recruitment to the complex.
   3. CD28 coreceptor binding to its ligand, B7 on dendritic cells, recruits PLCγ to the cell membrane.
   4. TCR ligation in the absence of coreceptor signaling can lead to **anergy** (unresponsiveness) in T cells.
      a. Clonal anergy is important in maintaining unresponsiveness to certain self antigens (Chapter 16).
      b. Conversely, the loss of clonal anergy among T cells that bear receptors for autoantigens can result in autoimmunity.

IV. The functions of antigen-activated T cells emerge after several cycles of cell division and differentiation.

   A. Most activated CD4$^+$ T cells express helper activity by secreting cytokines that act on other immune system cells.
   1. The CD4$^+$ T helper population can be further subdivided into the Th1 and Th2 cell subsets based upon the cytokines they secrete (Table 6–4 and Figure 6–5).

Table 6–4. Th1 and Th2 CD4$^+$ T cell subsets.[a]

Cytokine	Th1 Cells	Th2 Cells	Principal Functions
IL-2	++	−	Lymphocyte proliferation
IFN-γ	++	−	Macrophage activation Inhibition of IL-4 effects
LT (TNF-β)	++	−	Cytotoxicity
GM-CSF	++	+	Monocyte and dendritic cell differentiation
IL-4	−	++	B cell activation; Ig class switching; mast cell growth; inhibition of Th1 pathway
IL-5	−	++	B cell activation; Ig class switching; eosinophil growth and differentiation
IL-10	−	++	Inhibition of macrophage and lymphocyte activation
IL-13	−	++	Induction of mucus secretion; inhibition of IFN-γ action

[a]IL, interleukin; IFN, interferon; LT, lymphotoxin; TNF, tumor necrosis factor; GM-CSF, granulocyte macrophage colony-stimulating factor; Ig, immunoglobulin.

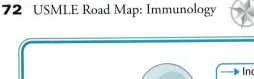

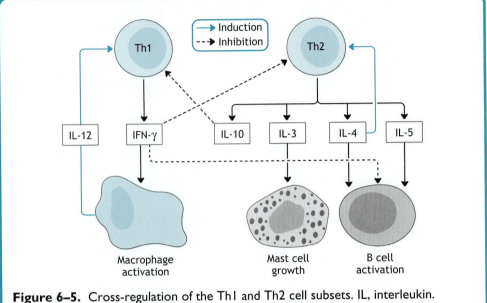

Figure 6–5. Cross-regulation of the Th1 and Th2 cell subsets. IL, interleukin.

    a. The **Th1 cell** subset produces cytokines primarily associated with **cell-mediated immunity** (ie, cytotoxic T cell growth and macrophage activation).
    b. The **Th2 cell** subset produces cytokines primarily associated with **humoral immunity** (ie, B cell activation, proliferation, differentiation, and Ig class switching).
  2. Some of the cytokines produced by the two Th cell subsets promote the development of their respective subset.
    a. IL-4 is an important inducer of the Th2 response.
    b. IFN-γ favors the development of a Th1 response.
  3. Each subset produces at least one cytokine that inhibits the functions of the other subset pathway (Figure 6–5).
    a. IL-10 and IL-4 produced by Th2 cells inhibit IL-12 production by APCs.
    b. IL-4 antagonizes the macrophage-activating effects of IFN-γ.
    c. IFN-γ produced by Th1 cells inhibits the proliferation of the Th2 cell subset.
    d. IFN-γ antagonizes the B cell-activating effects of IL-4.
  4. Dedicated transcription factors mediate the genetic control of Th1/Th2 development.
    a. **T-bet** is activated by IFN-γ and promotes Th1 cell development.
    b. **GATA-3** favors the development of a Th2 cell response.
B. Several populations of T cells express cytotoxic activity against foreign target cells (Table 6–5).
  1. Conventional CD8⁺ **cytotoxic T lymphocytes (CTL)** kill targets expressing foreign peptides and MHC class I molecules.
  2. Some CD4⁺ T cells are cytotoxic for targets expressing foreign peptides and MHC class II molecules.

Table 6–5. Cytotoxic lymphocytes.[a]

Property	CTL	NKT Cell	NK Cell
Receptors	TCRαβ; TCRγδ	Invariant TCRαβ	a
Receptor ligands	Peptides + MHC class I	Lipids and glycolipids + CD1	a
Surface markers	CD8 > CD4	CD8, CD4, and NK cell markers	NK cell markers (eg, CD161)
Functions	Cytotoxicity and cytokine production	Cytotoxicity and cytokine production	Cytotoxicity and cytokine production
Pathogens recognized	Viruses and intracellular bacteria	Unknown	Viruses

[a]For a description of the diverse NK cell receptors and their ligands, see Chapter 10. CTL, cytotoxic T cells; NKT, natural killer T; NK, natural killer; TCR, T cell receptor.

3. iNKT cells are cytotoxic against cells expressing glycolipid antigens presented by CD1 molecules.
4. All of these cytotoxic T cells require direct contact with their target cells and induce death by apoptosis (Figure 6–6).
   a. CTL reorient their killing components toward the cellular pole in contact with their target cell.
   b. Membrane-bound cytosolic **granules** of the cytotoxic cell then fuse with the cell membrane.
      (1) **Perforin** is a granule protein that polymerizes in the target cell membrane and facilitates the delivery of granzymes.
      (2) **Granzymes** are serine proteases that cleave caspases and initiate apoptosis in the target cell.
   c. **Fas ligand**, which is expressed on activated T cells and NKT cells, can induce apoptosis.
      (1) Fas ligand binds to a widely distributed receptor called **Fas**.
      (2) Fas contains death domains that recruit and activate the cytosolic caspases within the target cell.
   d. Cytotoxic cells secrete TNF-α and **lymphotoxin (LT)**, which bind to **TNF receptors**.
      (1) TNF receptors contain death domains that recruit adaptor proteins and activate caspases.
      (2) TNF receptors can also activate transcription factors that regulate gene expression (Chapter 12).
5. After delivering a lethal hit, the cytotoxic cell dissociates from its target cell and repeats the process with another target cell.

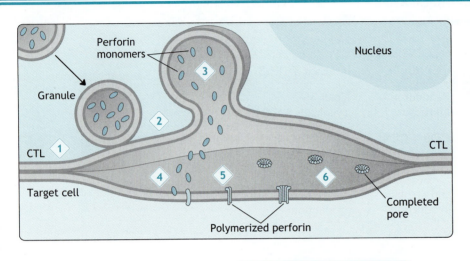

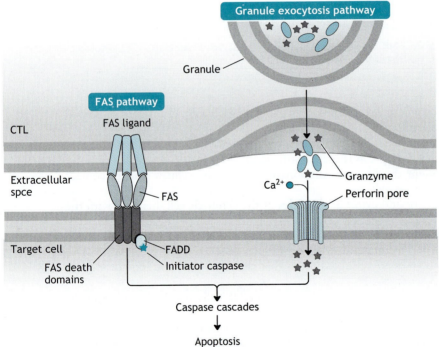

Figure 6–6. Conjugate formation and cell-mediated lysis by a cytotoxic T cell (CTL). (1) CTL-target cell contact, (2) granule fusion, (3) degranulation, (4) perforin insertion into target cell membrane, (5) polymerization of perforin, (6) pore formation

CLINICAL PROBLEMS

Infection of cells with certain herpes viruses leads to a decrease in the expression of class I MHC molecules by the infected cells.

1. For which of the following cytotoxic cells would this *decrease* its ability to recognize the virus-infected cell?

    A. CD4⁺ T cell

    B. CD8⁺ T cell

    C. NK cell

    D. NKT cell

    E. NK and NKT cell

A patient in renal failure received a kidney transplant from an unrelated donor. The patient was treated immediately with cyclosporine. Three weeks posttransplant, he developed an infection with cytomegalovirus that was attributed to his immunosuppressive therapy.

2. A decrease in which of the following responses would best explain this type of opportunistic infection?

    A. Transcriptional activation in B cells

    B. Ca^{2+} mobilization in macrophages

    C. Cytokine gene expression in T cells

    D. Neutrophil chemotaxis

    E. Signaling through the BCR

Ronald is a 2-year-old boy who presents with a 1-year history of recurrent sinus infections caused by gram-positive bacteria, including Group A streptococci. He has not had infections with viruses or fungi. He was successfully treated with antibiotics in the past, but his infections often returned after treatment ended. Laboratory tests indicate an elevated titer of anti-A and anti-B isohemagglutinins, but an IgG level that is less than 5% of the normal level for his age.

3. Which of the following mechanisms or diseases would be most consistent with this clinical picture?

    A. Bruton's X-linked agammaglobulinemia

    B. A deficiency of ZAP-70

    C. DiGeorge syndrome

    D. A lack of CD154 expression

    E. HIV-1 infection

Mary is an 11-year-old child with asthma. Allergy skin testing has revealed allergic reactions to 10 different household and outdoor allergens.

4. If you were to design an experimental therapy directed at reducing cytokine production in this disease, which of the following cytokines would be the best target of this therapy?

A. IL-1

B. IL-2

C. IL-4

D. IL-8

E. IL-12

A patient with recurrent viral infections has normal numbers of blood lymphocytes, but the cells do not express granzymes when activated in vitro.

5. A mutation in the gene encoding which of the following signaling intermediates would produce this phenotype?

A. Lck

B. Fas

C. MyD88

D. ZAP-70

E. Btk

ANSWERS

1. The correct answer is B. Among the choices, only CD8$^+$ T cells require MHC class I molecules for their recognition of viral peptide antigens. The expression of this protein can be inhibited by viruses that interfere with the synthesis of β_2-microglobulin, which is shared by MHC class I and CD1 molecules (Chapter 7).

2. The correct answer is C. Cyclosporine inhibits the phosphatase calcineurin, which is important in activating the transcription factor NFAT. NFAT regulates a number of cytokine genes in T cells, including those that coinduce virus-specific CD8$^+$ cytotoxic T cells to differentiate (eg, IL-2).

3. The correct answer is D. Elevated IgM antibody together with very low or absent IgG is an indication that the patient's B cells do not switch Ig class efficiently. This is typical of hyper IgM syndrome type 1, the congenital absence of CD154. The patient does not lack B cells, but fails to receive the proper signal from Th cells.

4. The correct answer is C. IL-4 plays a central role in the development of allergy by promoting Ig class switching to IgE and inducing more Th2 helper cells that produce IL-4. Mast cells are the source of inflammatory mediators in asthma, and their growth is also promoted by IL-4 (Chapter 13).

5. The correct answer is D. ZAP-70 deficiency causes a decreased signaling in both CD4$^+$ and CD8$^+$ T cells. Granzyme expression is a marker for activated cytotoxic lymphocytes.

CHAPTER 7
MAJOR HISTOCOMPATIBILITY COMPLEX

I. The principal function of the major histocompatibility complex (MHC) of genes is to regulate antigen recognition by T cells.

  A. In the thymus, MHC molecules determine the content of the T cell receptor (TCR) repertoire.

  1. Clones of thymocytes expressing TCRs that recognize foreign peptide antigens presented by the host's own MHC molecules are retained (Chapter 10).

  2. Clones of thymocytes with TCRs that recognize peptide antigens presented by nonhost MHC molecules are deleted.

  3. Mature thymocytes leave the thymus bearing TCRs capable of recognizing foreign peptides + self MHC in the periphery.

  B. In the postthymic environment, the MHC controls antigen recognition by mature T cells.

  1. The TCR recognizes antigenic peptides in the periphery only when they are complexed with a self MHC molecule.

    a. Antigen recognition by T cells is "MHC restricted."

    b. The TCR has a dual specificity for "altered self" (ie, self MHC + a foreign peptide).

  2. MHC genes are **immune response genes** that determine the magnitude of T cell activation by foreign protein antigens.

  C. MHC genes control the activation of natural killer (NK) cells by two mechanisms (Chapter 10).

  1. MHC gene products present peptides to NK cell **activating receptors**.

  2. MHC glycoproteins are also recognized by **inhibitory receptors** that suppress NK cell activation.

  D. The MHC serves as the most important genetic barrier to organ transplantation between two unrelated individuals of a species.

  1. In organ transplantation, the MHC molecules on a donor's tissues can be viewed by the recipient's T cells as foreign.

    a. In this context MHC molecules are **alloantigens**, antigens expressed by some, but not all, members of a species.

    b. MHC alloantigens stimulate vigorous T cell responses leading to graft rejection (Chapter 17).

II. MHC genes encode two classes of polypeptides that control antigen recognition by T cells.

A. MHC class I gene products present foreign peptides to CD8+ T cells.

1. Antigen recognition by CD8+ T cells is restricted by MHC class I molecules.
2. Only peptides bound to MHC class I molecules activate CD8+ T cells.
3. The three MHC class I genetic loci in human beings are called *human leukocyte antigen-A (HLA-A), HLA-B,* and *HLA-C.*
4. Each HLA class I gene encodes an ~45-kDa α polypeptide chain.
   a. Class I α chains are always expressed on the cell surface noncovalently associated with a 12-kDa invariant chain called **β₂-microglobulin** (Figure 7–1).
   b. Class I α chains are integral membrane proteins with three external domains.
      (1) Amino acids within the membrane-distal α1 and α2 domains are highly variable.

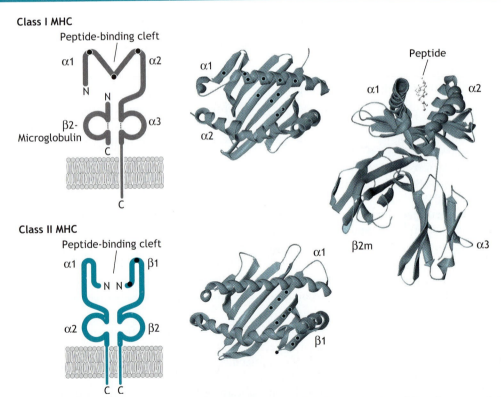

Figure 7–1. Structure of major histocompatibility complex (MHC) molecules. β2m, β₂-microglobulin. (Top: Adapted, with permission, from Bjorkman PJ: Structure of the human class I histocompatibility antigen, HLA-A2. Nature 1987;329:506.) (Bottom: Adapted, with permission, from Brown JH: Three-dimensional structure of the human class II histocompatibility antigen HLA-DR1. Nature 1993;364:33.)

(2) The α1 and α2 domains determine the peptide-binding specificity and alloantigenicity of class I.

(3) The membrane proximal α3 domain and β₂-microglobulin stabilize the overall structure.

5. MHC class I molecules possess a single **peptide-binding groove** within the α1 and α2 domains (Figure 7–1).

a. Contact residues within the groove determine specificity.

b. The typical peptide that binds to a class I molecule is 9–11 amino acids in length.

c. MHC class I-binding peptides contain terminal hydrophobic residues that anchor them into the groove.

d. Each MHC class I molecule shows **"promiscuous binding"** in that it can bind several different peptides.

B. The principal function of **MHC class II molecules** in the periphery is to present peptide antigens to CD4⁺ T cells.

1. Antigen recognition by CD4⁺ T cells is MHC class II restricted.

2. Only foreign peptides bound to MHC class II molecules can activate CD4⁺ T cells.

3. The MHC class II genes in human beings are found in three genetic regions called ***HLA-DP, HLA-DQ,*** and ***HLA-DR.***

4. Each class II genetic region contains one or more α and β genes.

a. The class II α and β loci encode for 33- and 28-kDa polypeptide chains, respectively.

b. The class II molecules form αβ heterodimeric cell surface glycoproteins (Figure 7–1).

c. Each chain has a membrane-distal domain (ie, α1 or β1) that is highly variable.

d. The α1 and β1 domains of class II molecules contain the peptide-binding groove.

e. These regions of sequence variability also prescribe the alloantigenic nature of class II molecules.

5. The peptide-binding groove of a typical class II molecule is similar in structure to that of a class I molecule.

a. Contact residues in the binding groove determine binding specificity.

b. MHC class II molecules typically bind 12–15 amino acid peptides that can extend beyond the limits of the groove.

c. Like class I, class II molecules show binding promiscuity.

C. Class I and class II MHC genes belong to the Ig supergene family.

D. MHC class III genes do not control T cell activation directly.

1. Class III genes include those for the complement proteins C2, C4, and Factor B (Chapter 8).

2. The gene for tumor necrosis factor (TNF)-α is also found in the class III MHC family.

ALTERED MHC-BINDING PEPTIDE LIGANDS

• *The nature of a T cell response to a peptide antigen can be altered by changing only a few of the contact residues of the peptide that interact with the TCR.*

- These **altered peptide ligands** include "superagonistic" peptides that can enhance T cell activation, which would be useful in designing antitumor immunotherapy.
- Similarly, altered peptide ligands can theoretically be designed that would inhibit unwanted T cell activation, such as that seen in autoimmune diseases.

III. MHC molecules show extensive functional diversity due to polygeny and genetic polymorphism.

A. Polygeny refers to the existence of multiple genetic loci that have similar functions.

1. Three MHC class I gene loci, *HLA-A, HLA-B,* and *HLA-C,* control antigen presentation to CD8$^+$ T cells.

2. Many MHC class II genetic loci control antigen presentation to CD4$^+$ T cells (eg, *DPα1, DPα2, DPβ1,* and *DPβ2*).

3. The existence of multiple MHC gene products increases the number of foreign peptides that can be presented to T cells.

B. Polymorphism within the MHC refers to the existence of multiple **alleles** of a gene within a population (Table 7–1).

1. Each class I allele encodes an α chain.

2. Each class II allele encodes either an α or a β chain.

3. A diploid individual can express at most two allelic products at each MHC locus (ie, in the heterozygote).

4. The β$_2$-microglobulin gene is *not* polymorphic.

5. Polymorphism has a greater effect on HLA diversity within the species than within an individual (Table 7–2).

   a. Thus, in the human population there is the capacity to present an enormous number of antigenic peptides.

   b. Each individual of that population has a much narrower potential repertoire of MHC-encoded molecules.

C. HLA diversity is sufficient for recognizing most protein antigens.

1. Each allelic product (eg, HLA-A1) can bind multiple peptides.

2. Each cell expresses multiple allelic forms (Figure 7–2).

Table 7–1. Examples of polymorphism at the HLA loci.

MHC Class	HLA Locus	Number of Alleles
I	HLA-A	250
I	HLA-B	490
I	HLA-C	119
II	HLA-DPA1	20
II	HLA-DPB1	99
II	HLA-DQA1	22
II	HLA-DQB1	53
II	HLA-DRB1	315
II	HLA-DRB3	38

Table 7–2. The basis for diversity among immunoglobulins and MHC molecules.

Feature	Immunoglobulin Genes	MHC Genes
Repertoire of an individual	~10^4 genes; ~10^9 Igs	6 class I alleles 6 class II alleles
Repertoire of the species	~10^4 genes; ~10^9 Igs	> 400 class I alleles > 500 class II alleles

Diversity mechanisms	Large pools of germ-line
	    V, D, J segments
	Combinatorial joining of
	    V, D, J segments
	Imprecision in joining sites
	Nucleotide additions at
	    joining sites
	Somatic hypermutation
	Combinatorial association
	    of H and L polypeptides
		Heterozygosity
		Codominant expression
		Polygeny
		Polymorphism

3. Mounting a successful response to a limited number of antigenic epitope–MHC complexes is apparently adequate to protect the host.

IV. MHC genes are inherited as a closely linked group of loci and are codominantly expressed (Figure 7–3).

A. HLA class I loci are clustered at the 3′ end of the complex on chromosome 6.

1. Each class I locus encodes an α chain, which is paired with β₂-microglobulin prior to surface expression (Figure 7–4).

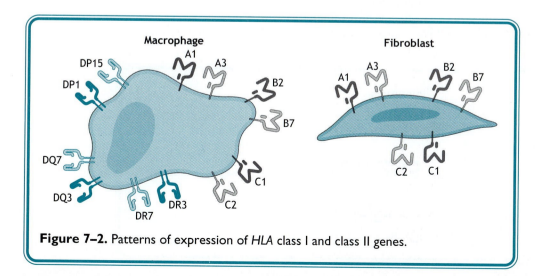

Figure 7–2. Patterns of expression of *HLA* class I and class II genes.

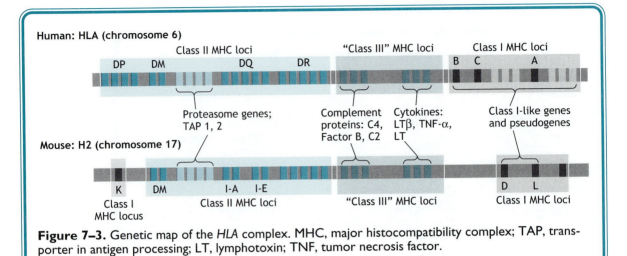

Figure 7–3. Genetic map of the *HLA* complex. MHC, major histocompatibility complex; TAP, transporter in antigen processing; LT, lymphotoxin; TNF, tumor necrosis factor.

 B. The class II loci are clustered at the 5′ end of the complex and code for either an α or a β chain.

  1. Different α and β gene products from a given region (eg, DP) can pair with one another to form heterodimeric products.

  2. Additional loci between the DP and DQ regions encode proteins that function in antigen presentation (see below).

 C. The closely linked genes of the MHC are inherited in a Mendelian fashion.

  1. The constellation of linked MHC genes on a given chromosome is called a **haplotype** (Table 7–3).

  2. Haplotype inheritance ensures that certain predictions can be made about HLA relationships within families (Figure 7–5).

   a. Assuming no genetic recombination has occurred, parents are always **haploidentical** with their children.

   b. Each child has a 75% chance of haploidentity with a sibling.

   c. Each child has a 25% chance of complete **HLA identity** with a sibling.

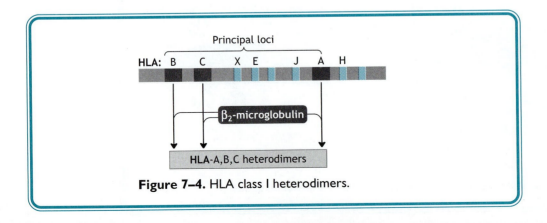

Figure 7–4. HLA class I heterodimers.

Table 7–3. Nomenclature of the HLA genetic system.

Term	Definition	Example
Region	A region within the HLA complex containing related genes	HLA-DR
Locus	An open reading frame that encodes for an HLA peptide	HLA-DRB1 (encodes a β chain of HLA-DR)
Allele	One of the alternative sequences at a locus	HLA-DRB1*0101
Antigen	A cell surface heterodimeric protein	HLA-DR1
Haplotype	The constellation of linked genes across the entire HLA complex on one chromosome	HLA-A1, B2, C5, DP2, DQ1, DR4

D. Individuals inherit parental MHC genes in their germ line DNA.
  1. The specificity of an individual's T cells is an inherited trait.
  2. The MHC loci do *not* rearrange prior to expression (Table 7–2).
E. MHC loci are expressed in a **codominant** fashion (Figure 7–2).
  1. All six allelic products of the HLA class I loci are expressed in the heterozygote.
    a. Each MHC class I heterodimer is expressed on all nucleated cells, except cells of the trophoblast.
    b. Any nucleated cell that expresses MHC class I molecules can present peptide antigens to CD8⁺ T cells.
    c. Each MHC class II heterodimer is expressed on all dendritic cells, B cells, and macrophages.
    d. Any such cell can present peptide antigens to CD4⁺ T cells.

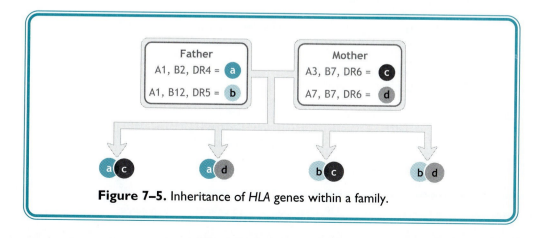

Figure 7–5. Inheritance of *HLA* genes within a family.

F. The expression of MHC class II genes is coordinately controlled by tissue-specific transcription factors, including the **class II transactivator (CIITA)**.
1. Constitutive expression of MHC class II is seen in B cells, monocytes, macrophages, and dendritic cells ("professional antigen-presenting cells").
2. Several other cell types (eg, epithelial cells) can be induced to express class II molecules by inflammatory signals.

COORDINATED EXPRESSION OF MHC CLASS II

- *An autosomal recessive condition expressed in infants called **bare lymphocyte syndrome (BLS) type 2** is characterized by lymphopenia, diarrhea, and a variety of opportunistic infections.*
- *These patients have significantly decreased numbers of blood CD4+ T cells, and show decreased cellularity in their peripheral lymphoid tissues.*
- *HLA-DP, DQ, and DR molecules are essentially absent from their tissues.*
- *In many BLS type II patients, the expression of CIITA is defective.*

V. **Two distinct pathways of antigen presentation ensure that foreign peptide antigens are presented by the proper MHC molecule to the appropriate T cell subset (Table 7–4 and Figure 7–6).**
A. **Intracellular microbes** (eg, viruses and intracellular bacteria) express protein antigens that are presented on class I molecules to CD8+ T cells.
1. Antigen presentation involves the degradation of these foreign proteins following their synthesis within the **cytosol**.
2. The resulting peptides are directed to newly synthesized class I molecules in the endoplasmic reticulum.

Table 7–4. Pathways of antigen processing and presentation.[a]

Pathway	Source of Antigen	Essential Cellular Components	Typical Antigens Processed
Class I	Endogenous	MHC class I α chains β₂-Microglobulin Ubiquitin Proteasome TAP-1,2 Chaperones (calnexin, tapasin, calreticulin)	Viral capsule proteins and nucleoproteins Proteins derived from intracellular bacteria
Class II	Exogenous	MHC class II α and β chains Ii chain CLIP HLA-DM	Proteins derived from extracellular pathogens Traditional protein vaccines

[a]TAP, transporter associated with antigen processing; CLIP, class II-associated invariant chain peptide.

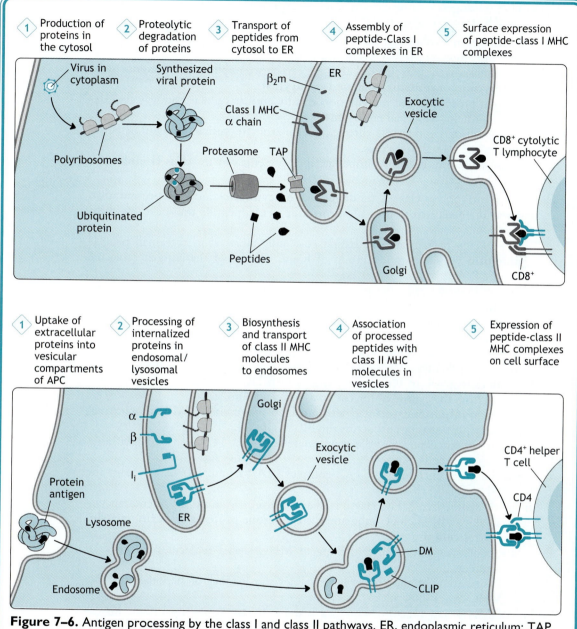

Figure 7–6. Antigen processing by the class I and class II pathways. ER, endoplasmic reticulum; TAP, transporter associated with antigen processing; MHC, major histocompatibility complex; CLIP, class II-associated invariant chain peptide.

3. These **endogenous protein antigens** are expressed on MHC class I and recognized by $CD8^+$ T cells.

B. **Extracellular microbes** activate $CD4^+$ T cells by expressing antigenic peptides that are presented on MHC class II molecules.
   1. The uptake of these exogenous antigens can be accomplished by **phagocytosis, endocytosis,** or **receptor-mediated endocytosis**.
   2. Antigen processing and presentation require an intracellular pathway that degrades proteins within an **endosome**.
   3. The resulting peptides are directed to an **exocytic vesicle** containing newly synthesized class II molecules.
   4. These exogenous protein epitopes are then presented by the **class II molecules** to $CD4^+$ T cells.

C. Components of the **class I (endogenous or cytosolic) antigen presentation pathway** are dedicated to proteolysis, peptide sizing, peptide transport, and protein targeting.
   1. The foreign protein antigen is first covalently attached to the small peptide **ubiquitin** via the ε-amino group of lysine residues of the antigen molecule (Figure 7–6).
   2. Ubiquitination targets the protein for degradation by the multicatalytic **proteasome**.
      a. The proteasome subunits LMP-2 and LMP-7, in part, determine substrate cleavage specificity.
      b. LMP-2 and LMP-7 are encoded by genes in the MHC (Figure 7–3).
      c. Peptides that leave the cylindrical proteasome vary in size and charge.
   3. Peptides that will fit the binding groove of MHC class I molecules are transported from the cytosol to the endoplasmic reticulum.
      a. The **transporter associated with antigen processing (TAP)** complex mediates peptide transport across the ER membrane.
      b. TAP selects peptides of the appropriate length (9–11 amino acids) with hydrophobic ends.
      c. The genes encoding the TAP complex, *TAP-1* and *TAP-2*, reside in the MHC (Figure 7–3).
   4. Newly synthesized MHC class I α chains are present in the ER membrane associated with $β_2$-microglobulin and the **chaperone proteins calnexin, tapasin, and calreticulum**.
      a. Chaperones direct the trafficking of MHC class I molecules to the TAP complex.
      b. Dissociation of the chaperones enables the loading of peptides into the MHC class I molecules.
   5. The MHC class I–peptide complex is then directed to the membrane for expression.
      a. The absence of $β_2$-microglobulin precludes surface expression of MHC class I molecules.
      b. The absence of a peptide in the binding groove of MHC class I prevents its surface expression.
      c. Pathogenic intracellular microbes often block the class I pathway by inhibiting $β_2$-microglobulin synthesis or TAP function.

6. In the absence of *foreign* antigenic peptides, MHC class I molecules are always loaded with *self* peptides.

BARE LYMPHOCYTE SYNDROME TYPE 1

- *Mutations in either the TAP1 or TAP2 gene prevent the transport of cytosolic peptides into the ER and result in incomplete peptide loading.*
- *Patients with these mutations do not express HLA-A, B, and C molecules on their nucleated cells, because class I molecules cannot be expressed unless they are loaded with peptide.*
- *These patients also fail to develop CD8+ T cells due to a defect in positive selection in the thymus (Chapter 10).*
- *The resulting immunodeficiency is not as severe as severe combined immunodeficiency (SCID), but can lead to opportunistic viral infections.*
- *Patients with BLS type 1 generally show normal numbers of circulating lymphocytes due to the normal development of the CD4+ T cell subset.*

  D. Peptides presented by MHC class II molecules are generally derived from extracellular proteins that are taken up by antigen-presenting cells.
  1. Following uptake into an endocytic or phagocytic vesicle, the organelle becomes increasingly acidic with time.
  2. Hydrolytic enzymes of the endolysosomes and phagolysosomes mediate proteolysis of the antigen.
  3. These vesicles then fuse with exocytic vesicles containing newly synthesized MHC class II molecules.
      a. Newly synthesized class II molecules are associated with a chaperone membrane protein called the **invariant chain (Ii)** .
      b. Ii ensures proper folding and protects the binding groove of the class II heterodimer.
  4. When the vesicles fuse, the Ii chain is degraded into a small peptide, called a **class II-associated invariant chain peptide (CLIP)**.
  5. **HLA-DM** catalyzes the removal of CLIP and the binding of appropriately sized antigenic peptides.
  6. The loaded MHC class II molecule is then directed to the cell surface.

VI. There are notable associations between specific HLA phenotypes and the susceptibility for certain diseases (Table 7–5).
  A. The relative risk of **hereditary hemochromatosis** is higher in individuals with the HLA-A3 + B14 haplotype than in the general population.
  1. Persons with this haplotype have an elevated incidence of mutations in a nonclassical MHC class I molecule called **HLA-H** (also known as HFE).
  2. HLA-H appears to regulate the function of the transferrin receptor, thereby affecting the absorption of dietary iron in the stomach and small intestine.
  3. Thus, certain mutations in HLA-H result in a chronic systemic exposure to excess iron resulting in hereditary hemochomatosis.
  B. HLA associations are particularly common among autoimmune diseases.
  1. **HLA-B27** expression is associated with an increased relative risk of **spondylarthropathies**.

Table 7–5. Disease associations with HLA phenotypes.

Disease	HLA Antigen or Haplotype	Relative Risk
Hereditary hemochromatosis	HLA-A3 + HLA-B14	90
Ankylosing spondylitis	HLA-B27	90
Reiter's syndrome	HLA-B27	37
Gluten enteropathy	HLA-DR3	12
Rheumatoid arthritis	HLA-DR4	14

  a. Spondylarthropathies are characterized by inflammation of the joints and characteristic extraarticular tissues.
  b. Individuals expressing HLA-B27 have an increased relative risk of developing the autoimmune conditions ankylosing spondylitis and Reiter's syndrome (Table 7–5).
  c. **Relative risk** is the prevalence of the disease in those carrying the HLA marker compared to the prevalence of the disease among the general population.
  d. A number of microbial antigens cross-react with HLA-B27–peptide complexes, suggesting an infectious etiology for these autoimmune diseases.

CLINICAL PROBLEMS

The HLA genetic system was used in a civil case to resolve a paternity suit. The case involved a woman who sued an acquaintance for child support for her newborn twins. The court ordered tissue typing (serological identification of the HLA markers; Chapter 17) of the mother, the two children, and the defendant. Partial results of the typing are shown below.

Individual	HLA-A Markers	HLA-B Markers
Mother	1,2	8,12
Son	1,3	8,7
Daughter	2,5	12,9
Defendant	3,3	7,28

1. Assuming there has been no recombination within the HLA complex, which haplotype did the son inherit from his mother?

A. HLA-A1 + HLA-A2

  B. HLA-A1 + HLA-B7

  C. HLA-A1 + HLA-B8

  D. HLA-A3 + HLA-B7

  E. HLA-B8 + HLA-B7

2. Assuming no recombination within the HLA complex, which haplotype did the daughter inherit from her mother?

  A. HLA-2 + HLA-B12

  B. HLA-2 + HLA-A5

  C. HLA-B12 + HLA-B9

  D. HLA-A2 + HLA-B9

  E. HLA-A5 + HLA-B12

3. Which of the following is a paternal haplotype that could have been inherited by one of the children from the defendant?

  A. HLA-A3 + HLA-B7

  B. HLA-A1 + HLA-B8

  C. HLA-A2 + HLA-B9

  D. HLA-A5 + HLA-B9

  E. HLA-A1 + HLA-B7

4. Based on these data alone, which of the following could be true?

  A. The son cannot be related to the defendant.

  B. The daughter cannot be related to the defendant.

  C. Neither child is related to the defendant.

  D. Both children could be related to the defendant.

  E. The two children have different fathers.

Below is a pedigree showing the HLA phenotypes of the Smith family. This is the second marriage for both the father and the mother.

5. Which of the five children shown here is most likely the child of a previous marriage involving the mother?

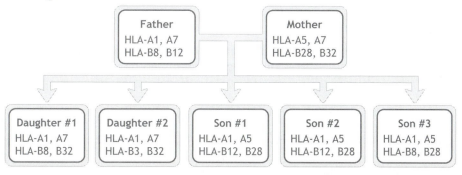

James is a 13-year-old child in need of a kidney transplant. He is the third of 14 children all with the same parents.

6. What are the chances that one of his siblings will be fully HLA compatible with James?

    A. There is almost no chance this will occur.

    B. 1 chance in 13

    C. 1 chance in 4

    D. 1 chance in 2

    E. All of his siblings would be HLA compatible.

ANSWERS

1. The correct answer is C. A haplotype is a group of linked genes (eg, HLA-A1 + HLA-B8) on one chromosome. In this case, the maternal haplotype can be derived by noting that these are the only HLA antigens shared between the mother and the son.

2. The correct answer is A. As with the son, these are the only HLA antigens shared with the mother. Thus, the son and daughter define the two maternal haplotypes, HLA-A1 + B8 and HLA-A2 + B12.

3. The correct answer is A. If A1, B8, A2, and B12 are of maternal origin, then the remaining HLA antigens were derived from the father. What is surprising in this case is that only the HLA-A3 + HLA-B7 haplotype is represented in the defendant's type.

4. The correct answers are B and E. Based on HLA typing it is safe to conclude that the daughter is *not* related to the defendant. Because these children are fraternal twins, it can only be concluded that the two children had different fathers. This is a case of apparent superfecundity, which occurs when two ova are produced during one ovulation cycle and become fertilized by sperm from two different fathers.

5. The correct answer is daughter #2. Analysis of the pedigree indicates that the haplotypes of the father are A1 + B8 and A7 + B12. The mother's haplotypes are A7 + B32 and A5 + B28. Daughter #2 bears the maternal haplotype A7 + B32, but the paternal haplotype does not correspond to those of the father. Therefore, the child must be from a previous marriage.

6. The correct answer is C. Based on Medelian inheritance in a codominant system, there is a 25% chance of full haplotype identity between siblings, assuming no recombinations or mutations.

CHAPTER 8
COMPLEMENT

I. Complement is a primitive immune effector and amplification system consisting of more than two dozen serum proteins.

    A. Complement components are designated by a **"C"** followed by a number (eg, C1) or the word **"Factor"** followed by an upper case letter (eg, Factor B).

    B. The **biological functions** of complement include cell membrane lysis, opsonization, activation of inflammatory responses, clearance of immune complexes, and B cell activation.

        1. Many of the biological activities are mediated by cell surface **complement receptors**.

        2. The complement system can be activated during either innate or adaptive immune responses.

    C. Complement system proteins become enzymatically or biologically active when they are cleaved, form multimers, or bind to other biomolecules.

II. The complement system can be activated by three different pathways (Table 8–1).

    A. In each pathway, complement is activated by the recognition of molecular patterns, on either antibody molecules or microbial components.

    B. All three activation pathways share a set of **core elements** that includes C3, C5, and the so-called **terminal components** C6–C9 (Figure 8–1).

        1. Initiation of each of the pathways requires recruitment or assembly of a serine protease.

        2. The critical second step is the cleavage of C3 by **C3 convertase** to form the peptide fragments C3a + C3b.

        3. Then C5 is cleaved by a **C5 convertase**.

        4. **Amplification** at each step results from the cleavage of multiple substrate molecules by these two convertases.

    C. The three pathways can be distinguished by their processes of initiation, their unique components, their unique functions, and the manner by which they are regulated (Table 8–1).

    D. The **classical pathway of complement activation** is initiated by antigen–antibody complexes.

        1. Only immunoglobulin (Ig) M and IgG antibodies participate in classical pathway activation.

Table 8–1. Three pathways of complement activation.[a]

Property	Classical Pathway	Lectin Pathway	Alternative Pathway
Initiating factors	IgG- or IgM-containing immune complexes	Microbial mannose residues	Highly charged surfaces
Unique components	C1, C2, C4	MBL, MASP	Factor B, Factor D, Factor P, Factor H
C3 convertase	C4b2a	C4b2a	C3bBb
C5 convertase	C4b2a3b	C4b2a3b	C3bBb3b
Unique functions	Adaptive immunity	Innate immunity	Innate immunity; positive feedback amplification; C3 tickover function
Unique regulators	C1 Inh		Factor H

[a]Ig, immunoglobulin; MBL, mannose-binding lectin; MASP, MBL-associated serine protease; C1 Inh, C1 inhibitor.

    2. Activation begins with the binding of the **C1q** peptide to the C_H domains of μ and γ heavy chains (Figure 8–2).
        a. C1q is a hexamer that cross-links two adjacent binding sites located on the C_H domains of μ or γ Ig heavy chains.
        b. IgM antibodies are more efficient than IgG antibodies in binding C1q, because the pentameric nature of IgM ensures that two C_H domains will be in close proximity to one another.

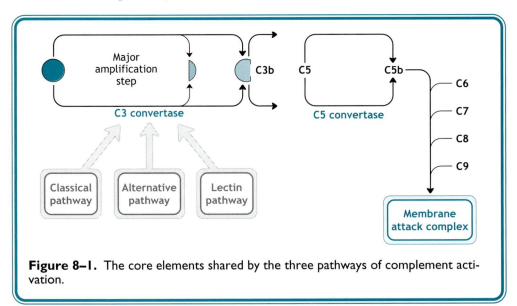

Figure 8–1. The core elements shared by the three pathways of complement activation.

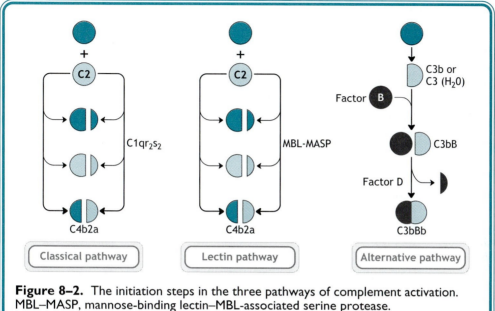

Figure 8–2. The initiation steps in the three pathways of complement activation. MBL–MASP, mannose-binding lectin–MBL-associated serine protease.

3. Once bound, C1q recruits two copies each of **C1r** and **C1s** to form an active enzyme.
4. The **C1qr$_2$s$_2$** complex can cleave C4 to yield peptides C4a and C4b.[1]
5. C1qr$_2$s$_2$ then cleaves C2 to yield the C2a + C2b peptides.
   a. C2a binds to C4b to produce C4b2a, the **classical C3 convertase**.
   b. This enzyme complex can cleave C3 to yield C3a + C3b.
6. Multiple copies of peptides are produced at each cleavage step.

HEREDITARY ANGIOEDEMA

- **Hereditary angioedema** *is a autosomal dominant trait characterized by acute, nonpainful, nonpruritic, and nonerythematous swelling of the skin and mucous membranes.*
- *Edema of the bowel wall can be painful, and laryngeal swelling is potentially life-threatening due to asphyxiation.*
- *The genetic defect is a decrease or absence of the complement regulatory protein, **C1 Inhibitor (C1 Inh)**, that regulates C1qr$_2$s$_2$, Hageman factor, kallikrein, and plasmin.*
- *Unabated complement activation through the classical pathway appears to contribute to the acute angioedema, although the precise biochemical mediator has not been defined.*

    E. The **lectin pathway of complement activation** shares properties and components with the classical pathway (Figure 8–2).

---

[1]A common convention in the complement field is the use of an overbar to designate enzymatically active complement components or complexes (eg, C1$\overline{qr_2s_2}$ or C$\overline{4b2a}$). For simplicity, this convention has been omitted here.

1. Activation is initiated by the binding of **mannose-binding lectin (MBL)** to microbial carbohydrate residues.
   a. MBL is another name for **mannose-binding protein** (Chapter 1).
   b. MBL recruits and binds **MBL-associated serine protease (MASP)**, an enzyme with substrate specificity similar to that of $C1qr_2s_2$.
2. MASP cleaves C4 and C2 to form the **lectin pathway C3 convertase**, C4b2a.

F. The **alternative pathway of complement activation** is initiated by at least three different mechanisms (Figure 8–2).
   1. Highly charged microbial surface patterns, including polysaccharides, can bind C3.
   2. In fluid phase, C3 can spontaneously hydrolyze with water to form an intermediate designated $C3(H_2O)$.
   3. The C3b peptide, derived from the classical or lectin pathways, can activate the alternative pathway directly.
   4. Bound C3, $C3(H_2O)$, or C3b then binds **Factor B**.
   5. Bound B is then cleaved by the constitutively active enzyme **Factor D** to produce Ba + Bb.
   6. C3Bb, $C3(H_2O)$Bb, and C3bBb are the **alternative pathway C3 convertases**.
      a. Whereas $C3(H_2O)$Bb is unstable, the other two complexes are relatively stable.
      b. C3bBb can be further stabilized by binding **Factor P**.
   7. The ability of the alternative pathway C3 convertases to generate more C3b constitutes a **feedback amplification loop** (Figure 8–3).

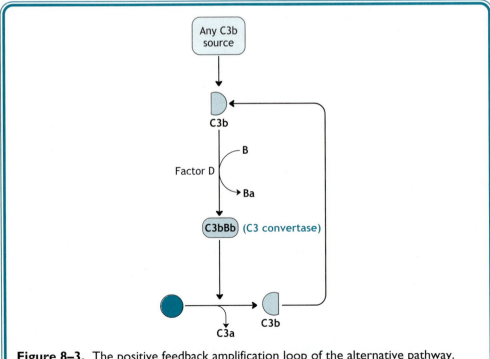

Figure 8–3. The positive feedback amplification loop of the alternative pathway.

8. Another unique feature of the alternative pathway is called **C3 tickover**.
  a. C3 constantly interacts with H_2O in fluid phase to form $C3(H_2O)$, an initiator of alternative pathway activation.
  b. However, the $C3(H_2O)$ intermediate is very unstable.
G. The peptides C3b and C4b can establish stable sites for further complement activation by covalently binding to appropriate surfaces.
  1. C3b and C4b contain internal **thioester bonds** that can be rearranged to form ester or amide linkages with biomolecules.
  2. These sites also provide covalently attached ligands for complement receptors.

III. The terminal steps in complement activation are shared by the three pathways.

A. C3 convertases are converted to **C5 convertases** by the binding of C3b (Table 8–1).
B. The C5 convertases cleave C5 generating C5a + C5b.
  1. **C5a** is a biologically active peptide that mediates chemotaxis and mast cell activation (see below).
  2. **C5b** is the first component of the **membrane attack complex (MAC)** (Figure 8–4).
    a. The assembly of the MAC does not require proteolysis.
    b. The assembled C5b678 complex can intercalate into the lipid membranes of both microbial and host cells.
    c. The C5b678 complex recruits multiple copies of C9 to form a stable membrane pore.
    d. Membrane disruption and rapid cell lysis result.

IV. The activation of complement is controlled at several levels (Table 8–2).

A. Some regulatory elements **inhibit** the formation of or **dissociate** active enzyme complexes.
  1. Many such inhibitors (eg, C1 Inh and **C4b-BP**) block early pathway initiation.
  2. Other inhibitors prevent the inadvertent lysis of host cells.
  3. Components, such as **HRF, CD59**, or **decay accelerating factor (DAF)**, are species specific and block complement activation on host, but not microbial, membranes.

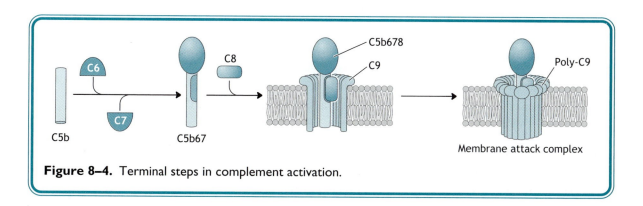

Figure 8–4. Terminal steps in complement activation.

Table 8–2. Regulation of the complement system.

Regulator	Pathway Affected	Mechanism of Action
C1 inhibitor (C1 Inh)	Classical	A serine protease inhibitor that dissociates $C1r_2s_2$ from C1q
C4b-binding protein (C4bBP)	Classical	Prevents formation of the classical and lectin pathway C3 convertase by blocking binding of C4b to C2a
CR1	All	Prevents formation of C3 convertases by blocking the binding of C3b to Factor B or the binding of C4b to C2a
Factor P	Alternative	Stabilizes C3bBb
Factor H	Alternative	Blocks formation of C3bBb by binding to C3b
Decay accelerating factor (DAF)	All	Accelerates the decay of the C3 convertases C4b2a and C3bBb
Factor I	All	Cleaves C3b and C4b to produce iC3b and iC4b, respectively
Anaphylatoxin inhibitor (AI)	All	Cleaves and inactivates the anaphylatoxins C3a, C4a, and C5a
S protein	All	Prevents membrane insertion of the C5b67 complex
Hemologous restriction factor (HRF)	All	Prevents binding of poly-C9 to the C5b678 complex

   B. Several regulatory factors **inactivate** biologically active complement peptides by proteolysis.
   1. **Anaphylatoxin inhibitor (AI)** cleaves the terminal arginine residues of peptides C3a, C4a, and C5a, rendering them inactive.
   2. **Factor I** cleaves C3b and C4b, destroying their ability to form C3 convertases.
   C. Some factors (eg, S protein) prevent membrane attack by **blocking the assembly** of a mature MAC.

TRANSGENIC PIGS, MEMBRANE ATTACK, AND XENOTRANSPLANTATION

• The worldwide shortage of organs suitable for clinical transplantation has stimulated research on the transplantation of organs between species (**xenotransplantation**).

- *The early rejection of xenografts, including pig grafts in human beings, appears to be mediated by natural human antibodies and complement.*
- *The membranes of pig cells appear to be particularly susceptible to membrane attack, because their complement regulatory proteins do not inhibit human complement components (eg, C3 convertases and MAC).*
- *A novel approach to this dilemma has been to create transgenic pigs expressing human complement regulatory proteins (eg, DAF).*
- *If successful, these animals could be developed as a source of organs for clinical transplantation.*

V. The biological activities of the complement system depend on the action of its peptides and assembled complexes (Table 8–3).

A. Membrane damage is caused by the assembly of the **MAC** in a lipid bilayer.
1. This is an important mechanism of host cell lysis in transfusion reactions, transplantation rejection, and autoimmunity.
2. The MAC can lyse the exposed outer membranes of Gram-negative bacteria.
3. Membrane damage caused by MAC is similar to that caused by perforin produced by cytotoxic T cells (Chapter 6).
   a. Poly-C9 and poly-perforin produce membrane pores.
   b. Perforin and C9 show considerable amino acid sequence homology.

FACTOR I DEFICIENCY

CLINICAL CORRELATION

- *Because Factor I destroys C3 convertases by cleaving C3b and C4b, it regulates complement activation at a key amplification step.*
- *The importance of **Factor I** in this regard is illustrated by individuals with hereditary Factor I deficiency.*

Table 8–3. Summary of important complement components and complexes.[a]

	Classical Pathway	Lectin Pathway	Alternative Pathway
Enzymatic components	$C1qr_2s_2$ C4b2a C4b2a3b	MBL-MASP C4b2a C4b2a3b	Factor D C3bBb C3bBb3b
Biologically active peptides or complexes	C3b C4b C3d C3a C4a C5a $C5b-9_n$	C3b C4b C3d C3a C4a C5a $C5b-9_n$	C3b C4b C3d C3a C4a C5a $C5b-9_n$
Important regulatory components	C1 Inh C4b-BP Factor I	C4b-BP Factor I	Factor P Factor I Factor H

[a]MBL-MASP, mannose-binding lectin-MBL-associated serine proteases; C1 Inh, C1 inhibitor; C4b-BP, C4b binding protein.

• *These patients suffer from recurrent pyogenic infections, including meningococcal meningitis.*

• *The treatment of these patients with recombinant Factor I provides some relief during acute infections, but its long-term clinical effectiveness is unknown.*

    B. Many complement peptides exert their biological effects through cell surface **complement receptors (CR)** (Table 8–4).

      1. Complement receptor 1 (CR1) mediates the clearance of circulating immune complexes that bear C3b or C4b.

        a. Erythrocytes bear the highest densities of CR1 and mediate the greatest share of immune complex clearance.

        b. The complexes are delivered to the liver, where they are taken up by Kupffer cells.

      2. CR2 mediates B cell coactivation when C3d-coated antigens cross-link CR2 and BCR (Figure 8–5).

      3. The **opsonic** activity of C3b, iC3b, C4b, and iC4b is due to the binding of particles coated with these peptides to **CR1, CR3,** and **CR4.**

      4. The **C3a/4a receptor (CR3a/4aR)** mediates mast cell degranulation (Chapter 13).

      5. C5aR is a G protein-coupled seven transmembrane chemotactic receptor that mediates the chemoattraction of neutrophils.

    C. Microbes have developed elaborate mechanisms of immune evasion by targeting the complement system and diminishing its biological activities.

      1. Herpes simplex virus produces a glycoprotein (C) that promotes C3 decay.

Table 8–4. Complement receptors.

Complement Receptor	Ligands	Cell Expressing the Receptor	Principal Biological Activities
CR1	C3b, iC3b C4b, iC4b	Erythrocytes, phagocytic cells	Clearance of immune complexes
CR2	C3d	B cells	B cell coactivation
CR3	C3b, iC3b C4b, iC4b	Phagocytic cells	Immune complex binding, opsonophagocytosis, cell adhesion
CR4	C3b, iC3b C4b, iC4b	Phagocytic cells	Immune complex binding, opsonophagocytosis, cell adhesion
C3a/C4a R	C3a, C4a	Mast cells	Degranulation leading to inflammatory mediator release
C5aR	C5a	Neutrophils Mast cells	Chemotaxis Degranulation and mediator release

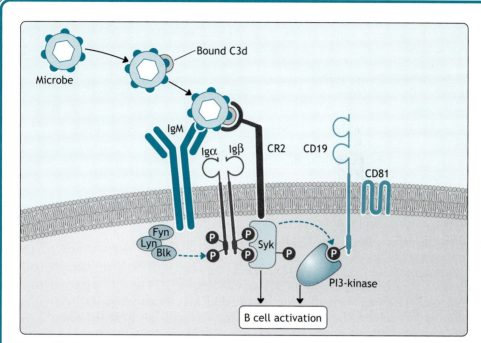

Figure 8–5. Signaling through the B cell coreceptor by binding C3d. Ig, immunoglobulin; PI3-kinase, phosphatidylinositol-3-kinase.

    2. The long, branching polysaccharide chains of bacterial surface lipopolysaccharides are thought to direct complement activation away from the outer lipid membrane (Figure 1–3).

    3. *Pseudomonas aeruginosa* produces a protease that cleaves C3b.

VI. Complement plays a central role in the pathogenesis of human disease.

    A. Serum complement levels can be markedly decreased in **immune complex diseases**.

        1. The circulating levels of C1, C2, C3, and C4 decline when immune complexes containing IgM or IgG antibodies activate the classical pathway.

            a. Total complement activity is measured in **complement hemolytic 50% (CH_{50}) units**.

            b. Standard CH_{50} assays measure the activity of the classical pathway.

        2. Regularly measuring total serum complement can be an effective means of monitoring the therapy of immune complex diseases.

    B. C3b often deposits within tissues and induces inflammation (Chapter 13).

    C. **Primary deficiencies of complement** components cause inflammatory and infectious diseases.

        1. Inherited deficiencies (generally autosomal recessive) of most of the individual complement components have been described.

2. Deficiencies of the early classical and alternative pathways (eg, C1, C2, C4, and Factor B) are most often associated with an increased risk of bacterial infections.
3. The absence of C9 has only a minimum effect on infection rates.
4. Patients with congenital deficiencies of C5, C6, C7, or C8 have an increased risk of disseminated *Neisseria* infections (eg, meningitis).
5. These observations would suggest that complement-dependent lysis of bacteria is *less* important to the host than is its role in the chemotaxis and opsonophagocytosis by neutrophils.

D. **Paroxysmal nocturnal hemoglobinuria (PNH)** is a condition characterized by episodes of intravascular hemolysis and hemoglobinuria.
   1. Patients' erythrocytes are particularly sensitive to complement-mediated lysis.
   2. PNH patients lack the GPI-linked membrane proteins DAF and CD59.
      a. Membrane C3 convertases are not well controlled, resulting in the deposition of C3b (Table 8–2).
      b. Assembly of the MAC is also not regulated at the cell membrane.

E. **Leukocyte adhesion defect type 1 (LAD-1)** is a deficiency in the expression of complement receptors CR3 and CR4.
   1. LAD-1 involves a mutation in the β_2 integrin CD18 (Table 8–5).
   2. **CD18** normally forms heterodimers with **CD11a, CD11b,** or **CD11c.**
      a. The CD11a–CD18 dimer is the adhesion molecule **LFA-1,** which facilitates neutrophil binding to endothelial cells and leukocyte emigration from the blood.
      b. The CD11b–CD18 and CD11c–CD18 dimers are **CR3** and **CR4,** respectively, which are adhesion and opsonic receptors on phagocytic cells.
   3. LAD-1 patients suffer from recurrent pyogenic infections.

COMPLEMENT DEFICIENCIES AND AUTOIMMUNITY

- *Patients with deficiencies of the early classical pathway components (eg, C2 and C4) have an increased incidence of autoimmune disorders, especially lupus-like nephritis.*
- *This may reflect their inability to clear immune complexes that contain C3b generated by the classical pathway.*
- *Conversely, patients with immune complex-mediated autoimmunity often show depressed levels of C1, C2, C3, and C4 during acute attacks.*
- *$C1qr_2s_2$, C4b, C2a, and C3b are removed from the circulation when immune complexes are cleared by CR1-expressing erythrocytes.*

Table 8–5. Leukocyte adhesion defect type 1.[a]

CD18 Heterodimeric Partner	Receptor Formed	Receptor Ligands
CD11a	LFA-1	ICAM-1
CD11b	CR3	iC3b, iC4b
CD11c	CR4	iC3b, iC4b

[a]LFA-1, lymphocyte function-associated antigen-1; ICAM-1, intercellular adhesion molecule 1.

CLINICAL PROBLEMS

A patient presents with recurrent joint pain and renal insufficiency, which is associated with immune complex deposition in these organs. It is determined that the patient does not clear IgG-containing immune complexes from the circulation at a normal rate.

1. A defect in which of the following complement receptors would most contribute to this latter finding?

A. CR1

B. CR2

C. CR3

D. CR4

E. CR5

Mary is a 2-year-old child with a history of recurrent upper respiratory tract infections. She has normal serum Ig levels for her age, and her complete blood count (CBC) and tests for neutrophil functions are normal. The total complement activity of her serum is normal in terms of supporting the lysis of antibody-coated erythrocytes. However, her serum complement is not activated by bacterial lipopolysaccharide (LPS).

2. Which of the following primary deficiencies of the complement system would be most consistent with these findings?

A. C2 deficiency

B. Factor D deficiency

C. MBL deficiency

D. C1 Inh deficiency

E. DAF deficiency

A 4-year-old child is referred to you with a diagnosis of leukocyte adhesion defect. She has a history of recurrent bacterial infections, including pneumonias and skin abscesses. Radiology demonstrates granuloma-like lesions in her lung and liver. However, the data in the table below suggest this condition has not been properly diagnosed.

3. Which element of the table is **inconsistent** with a diagnosis of LAD?

CD Marker	Patient (%)	Normal Range (%)
CD2	76	75–93
CD3	75	60–85
CD4	52	30–65
CD8	26	20–52
CD11a	65	62–85
CD18	73	70–86
CD19	12	7–17
CD45	52	44–62

A. CD2

B. CD3

C. CD19

D. CD11a

E. CD45

A pediatric patient presents with recurrent staphylococcal infections (pneumonias, sinusitis, and otitis media). Because many of her immune parameters are normal, you hypothesize that she has a defect in her complement system.

4. For which of the following complement components or receptors would a deficiency produce this pattern of recurrent infections?

A. C2

B. C6

C. C8

D. CR1

E. CD59

A patient with the immune complex autoimmune disease systemic lupus erythematosus (SLE) is experiencing significant symptoms, including a worsening of her skin rash and evidence of impaired renal function.

5. If you were to test her serum complement levels during this acute phase of disease, which of the following would be most consistent with a worsening clinical course?

A. A decline in C9 levels

B. A decline in C3 and C4 levels

C. An increase in Factor P levels

D. An increase in C1 Inh levels

E. A decline in C7 levels

ANSWERS

1. The correct answer is A. Complement receptor CR1 is responsible for clearing immune complexes from the circulation by binding to C3b or iC3b. While CR3 and CR3 show the same ligand specificity, the substantially larger number of CR1 receptors expressed by numerous erythrocytes in the blood make this receptor the primary vehicle of immune complex clearance.

2. The correct answer is B. Of the choices, only Factor D is unique to the alternative pathway of complement, which is activated by bacterial LPS. A deficiency of Factor D prevents cleavage of Factor B, which is essential for producing the alternative pathway C3 convertase.

3. The correct answer is D. This patient appears to express normal levels of all of the CD markers shown here. This would *not* be expected of a patient with LAD type 1. Such patients lack CD18, which impairs the expression of CD11a, CD11b, and CD11c.

4. The correct answer is A. Of the components listed, only deficiencies in C2, C6, and C8 result in an increased susceptibility to bacterial infections. With C6 and C8, the pathogens are members of the *Neisseria* genus and certain other gram-negative bacteria. Defects in early classical components, such as C2, result in recurrent pyogenic infections by gram-positive bacteria, such as staphylococci.

5. The correct answer is B. Lupus is an autoimmune disease in which complement is activated by IgG autoantibodies via the classical pathway. This can lead to an acute depletion in the early classical components, such as C1, C2, C3, and C4. The concentrations of the terminal components are affected much less.

CHAPTER 9
B CELL DIFFERENTIATION AND FUNCTION

I. The development of a diverse, self-tolerant population of antigen-specific B cells is central to creating an adaptive immune system.

A. The initial events of **lymphopoiesis** occur in the fetal liver and bone marrow and do not require exposure to foreign antigens.

1. **Hematopoietic stem cells (HSC)**, which express **CD34**, are **pluripotent** and can become any of the blood cell lineages (eg, erythroid, lymphoid, myeloid).

2. Lineage commitment is determined by the **hematopoietic inductive microenvironment**, which includes stromal cell ligands and growth factors (Chapter 12).

3. **Interleukin-7 (IL-7)** is an important growth factor for B and T lymphocyte development.

4. Lymphocyte lineage commitment is indicated by the formation of the **lymphoid progenitor cell.**

5. Commitment to the B lymphocyte lineage occurs at the **progenitor B (pro-B) cell** stage (Table 9–1).

   a. Most pro-B cells express **CD19** as do all subsequent cells of the B cell lineage.

   b. **Recombination activating genes 1 and 2 (Rag1, Rag2)** and **terminal deoxynucleotidyltransferase (TdT)** are expressed in preparation for immunoglobulin (Ig) locus rearrangements.

   c. The Ig H chain locus is rearranged by VDJ recombination, but H chain polypeptides are not expressed.

6. The pro-B cell differentiates into a **precursor-B (pre-B) cell**, which expresses a pre-B cell receptor (BCR).

   a. The **pre-BCR** consists of a membrane μ chain, an invariant **surrogate L chain,** and Igα and Igβ polypeptides.

   b. Signaling through the pre-BCR induces allelic exclusion at the Ig H locus and rearrangement of the κ locus.

7. The pre-B cell differentiates into an **immature B cell** expressing an authentic BCR.

   a. The BCR complex consists of membrane μ chains, κ or λ light chains, and the Igα and Igβ polypeptides.

   b. Immature B cells exit the bone marrow and complete their differentiation into mature B cells in the periphery.

   c. Most immature B cells die in the periphery unless they encounter antigen.

Table 9–1. Stages of antigen-independent B cell differentiation.[a]

	HSC	Pro-B	Pre-B	Immature B	Mature B
Igα, Igβ	–	+	+	+	+
Rag1, 2	–	+	+	+	–
TdT	–	+	+	–	–
Surrogate L chain	–	+	+	–	–
Membrane μ chain	–	–	+	+	+
Membrane δ chain				–	+
Membrane κ or λ chain	–	–	–	+	+
Btk kinase	–	+	+	+	+
Positive selection	-	–	+	+	–
Negative selection	–	–	–	+	–

[a]HSC, hematopoietic stem cells; Ig, immunoglobulin; Rag1, Rag2, recombination activating genes 1 and 2; Tdt, terminal deoxynucleotidyltransferase; Btk, Bruton's tyrosine kinase.

8. **Mature B cells** express two forms of the BCR, membrane IgM and membrane IgD (Chapter 4).
   a. **B-1 B cells** are among the first peripheral B cells and are found predominantly in the peritoneal and pleural cavities.
   b. B-1 B cells produce natural antibodies thought to be induced by microbial flora.
   c. B-1 B cells have a limited BCR repertoire.
      (1) Most B-1 B cells produce low-affinity IgM antibodies specific for **polysaccharide antigens**.
      (2) The BCRs of B-1 B cells contain relatively conserved V regions.
B. **Selection** occurs at several differentiation checkpoints and determines the peripheral B cell repertoire.
   1. **Positive selection** rescues bone marrow B cells from apoptosis ("death by neglect") (Table 9–2).
      a. Positive selection occurs at the pre-B and immature B cell stages.
      b. Selection requires signaling through the pre-BCR or BCR.
      c. The pre-BCR signals differentiation to the immature B cell stage and the BCR promotes differentiation into mature B cells.
      d. Positive selection through the BCR probably involves low affinity binding to self-ligands.

Table 9–2. Positive and negative selection of developing B cells.[a]

	Positive Selection	Negative Selection
Stage of B cell development	Pre-B cell Immature B cell	Immature B cell
Receptors	Pre-BCR BCR	BCR
Ligands	Unknown	Self antigens
Events triggered by selection	Allelic exclusion of H locus Proliferation of pre-B cells κ locus rearrangement	Apoptosis BCR editing Secondary κ locus rearrangement
Outcome	Advancement to immature B cell stage Monoclonal expression of μ chain BCR expression	Elimination of autoreactive B cell clones Replacement of autoreactive BCRs

[a]BCR, B cell receptor.

X-LINKED AGAMMAGLOBULINEMIA

- *X-linked agammaglobulinemia (XLA)* is a congenital immune deficiency characterized by the lack of peripheral B cells.
- *Agammaglobulinemia* becomes apparent only after maternal IgG disappears during the first year of life.
- XLA patients have a mutation in the gene coding for **Bruton's tyrosine kinase (Btk)**.
- Btk is first required for signaling by the pre-BCR at the pre-B cell stage and mediates positive selection.
- A similar phenotype exists in patients with H locus deletions that prevent functional μ chain synthesis and pre-BCR expression.

   2. **Negative selection** mediates removal of autoreactive B cell clones.
      a. Negative selection establishes **self-tolerance**.
      b. Negative selection occurs at the immature B cell stage and is mediated by high-affinity BCR binding of self antigens.
      c. Negative selection can signal either apoptosis or anergy within B cells.
      d. Negative selection can stimulate **BCR editing**.
         (1) The cell undergoes a second light chain locus rearrangement.

(2) The second rearrangement replaces the L chain of the self-reactive BCR.
(3) The B cell undergoes another round of selection based on its new BCR.

II. In the periphery, antigen induces further differentiation of mature B cells into antibody-producing plasma cells and memory cells.

A. Antigen enters the spleen, lymph nodes, and submucosal lymphoid follicles via the blood, the lymph, or by transport across the mucosal epithelium, respectively.

B. A single antigen-reactive B cell can give rise to thousands of daughter cells through 10--12 cell doublings.

C. Activated B cells differentiate into sessile **plasma cells** that live for only a few days.
   1. Differential RNA processing ensures that plasma cells synthesize secreted, rather than membrane, Igs (Chapter 4).
   2. The progeny of a single B cell can synthesize up to 10^{12} antibody molecules.

D. Antigen-specific, long-lived **memory B cells** also arise during B cell clonal expansion in lymph node **germinal centers.**
   1. **Follicular dendritic cells** promote memory B cell development by retaining antigens over long periods of time.
   2. Germinal center development is T cell dependent.
   3. Memory B cells undergo Ig isotype switching.
   4. Memory B cells mediate **secondary responses** characterized by the following:
      a. A requirement for less antigen to induce the response.
      b. A shorter lag period before antibody is detected.
      c. Higher average affinity of the antibodies produced.
      d. The presence of additional Ig isotypes.

E. **Affinity maturation** accompanies memory B cell development.
   1. Affinity maturation is an increase in the average affinity of an antibody response over time.
   2. Affinity maturation is T cell dependent.
   3. Affinity maturation requires **somatic hypermutation** of Ig V region genes.
      a. Proliferating B cell clones bear mutations in the complementarity determining regions of their BCRs.
      b. The average affinities of the antibodies these cells produce increase by 10- to 100-fold.
      c. Cells that express mutated, high-affinity BCRs are **positively selected** by antigen for additional cycles of proliferation.

III. Antigen-induced activation of B cells is mediated through the BCR, coreceptors, and cytokine receptors (Figure 9–1).

A. The BCRs on mature naive B cells are membrane IgM and IgD.

B. Memory B cells utilize membrane IgG, IgA, or IgE as their BCRs.

C. Each of these BCRs signals through Igα and Igβ and intermediates that are similar to those used by the T cell receptor (TCR) (Chapter 6) (Table 9–3).

D. Signaling is initiated by clustering of the BCR complex.
   1. Polyvalent antigens with repeating identical determinants can activate B cells without coreceptor signals.
   2. Most native protein antigens contain univalent epitopes that do not mediate BCR cross-linking.

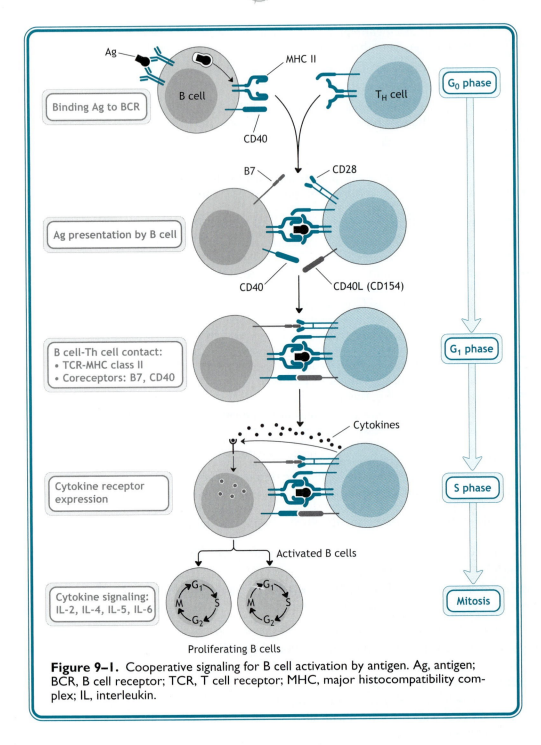

Figure 9–1. Cooperative signaling for B cell activation by antigen. Ag, antigen; BCR, B cell receptor; TCR, T cell receptor; MHC, major histocompatibility complex; IL, interleukin.

Table 9–3. Analogous components of the TCR and BCR signaling pathways.[a]

Signaling Event or Intermediate	TCR Associated	BCR Associated	Effects
Clustering of receptors in the membrane	TCRαβ or TCRγδ with CD3 peptides	BCR with Igα and Igβ	Concentrate subsequent signaling mediators
Phosphorylation of ITAMs	Phosphorylation of CD3 ITAMs by Lck	Phosphorylation of Igα and Igβ ITAMs by Src kinases	Binding sites for downstream adaptor proteins and kinases
Effector kinase recruitment and activation	ZAP-70	Syk	Phosphorylates downstream adapters and kinases
Phospholipase activation	PLCγ	PLCγ	PIP_2 hydrolysis
IP_3 and DAG	Ca^{2+} mobilization PKC activation	Ca^{2+} mobilization PKC activation	Calcineurin activation
Calcineurin activation	NFAT dephosphorylation	NFAT dephosphorylation	Transcriptional activation through NFAT
PKC activation of IκB kinase	IκB phosphorylation	IκB phosphorylation	Transcriptional activation through NFκB
Rac, Ras activation of MAP kinases	Fos/Jun phosphorylation	Fos/Jun phosphorylation	Transcriptional activation through NFκB

[a]TCR, T cell receptor; BCR, B cell receptor; Ig, immunoglobulin; ITAM, immunotyrosine activation motif; ZAP-70, ζ-associated protein-70 kDa; PLC, phospholipase C; PIP_2, phosphatidylinositol 4,5-biphosphate; IP_3, inositol triphosphate; DAG, diacylglycerol; PKC, protein kinase C; MAP, mitogen-activated protein.

3. Igα and Igβ transmit BCR signals across the cell membrane.
   a. The cytoplasmic domains of Igα and Igβ contain **immunotyrosine activation motifs (ITAM)** (Figure 9–2).
   b. **Src family kinases** phosphorylate ITAM tyrosine residues.
4. The tyrosine kinase **Syk** is recruited to the phosphorylated ITAMs, becomes phosphorylated, and phosphorylates downstream adapter proteins (eg, BLNK) and latent kinases.
   a. Btk kinase is recruited to BLNK and activates **phospholipase Cγ (PLCγ)**.
      (1) PLCγ hydrolyzes the membrane phospholipid phosphatidylinositol 4,5-biphosphate (PIP_2) to form inositol triphosphate (IP_3) and diacylglycerol (DAG).
      (2) IP_3 mobilizes intracellular Ca^{2+} and activates **calcineurin**.
      (3) Calcineurin activates the transcription factor **NFAT** by dephosphorylation.

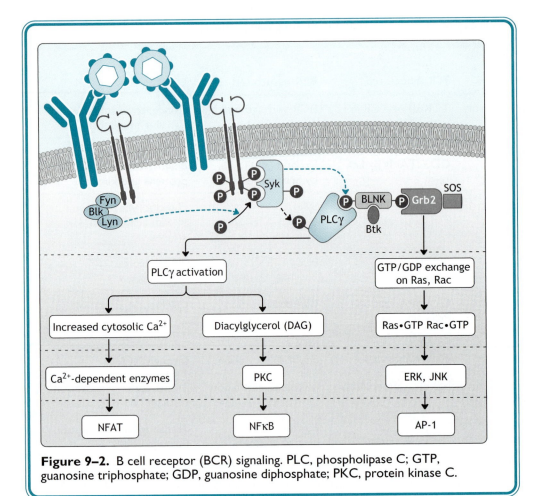

Figure 9–2. B cell receptor (BCR) signaling. PLC, phospholipase C; GTP, guanosine triphosphate; GDP, guanosine diphosphate; PKC, protein kinase C.

        (4) Protein kinase C is activated by DAG, which indirectly induces the degradation of **IκB**, the inhibitor of **NFκB**.

        (5) The transcription factor NFκB is activated.

    b. The guanosine triphosphate/guanosine diphosphate (GTP/GDP) exchange proteins **Rac** and **Ras** are activated.

        (1) Rac and Ras activate mitogen-activated protein (MAP) family kinases.

        (2) The MAP kinases activate the **AP-1** family of transcription factors (eg, Fos and Jun) by phosphorylation.

  5. NFAT, NFκB, and AP-1 translocate to the nucleus and initiate gene transcription by binding to their respective enhancers.

  6. The transcription of Ig, coreceptor, and cytokine receptor genes is initiated or increased.

E. Coreceptors enhance signals delivered through the BCR (Table 9–4).

  1. Contact with T helper cells is required for coreceptor signaling.

Table 9–4. Important receptors and coreceptors on B cells.[a]

Receptor or Coreceptor	Ligand	Biological Response
Pre-BCR	Unknown	Positive selection of pre-B cells
BCR	Self antigens	Positive and negative selection of immature B cells
	Foreign antigens	Activation of peripheral mature B cells
CR2	C3d	Coactivation of mature B cells Enhancement of BCR signaling
CD40	CD154 (CD40L)	Coactivation of mature B cells Enhancement of BCR signaling
IL-2R	IL-2	Growth of activated B cells
IL-4R	IL-4	Switching to IgE
IL-5R	IL-5	Switching to IgA
IL-6R	IL-6	Differentiation of cycling B cells Increased Ig synthesis
CCR7	CCL7	Chemotaxis of germinal center B cells

[a]BCR, B cell receptor; IL, interleukin; Ig, immunoglobulin.

   a. The chemokine **CCL7** mediates chemoattraction of B cells to the outer edge of germinal centers where they bind Th cells.
   b. Contact-dependent signaling is promoted by **major histocompatibility complex (MHC) class II,** on B cells, which is bound by the TCR.
   c. T cell contact-dependent signaling promotes B cell **proliferation,** increases **MHC class II** expression, induces **coreceptor, cytokine receptor,** and **chemokine receptor** expression, promotes **affinity maturation,** and induces **Ig class switching**.
2. **CD154** (CD40 ligand or CD40L) on CD4⁺ Th cells coactivates B cells by binding to CD40.
   a. **CD40** signals B cells to switch Ig class by H chain gene locus rearrangement.
   b. Mutations in the CD154 gene can block T cell-induced Ig class switching in B cells **(hyper-IgM syndrome type 1)**.
3. Complement activation during innate and adaptive immune responses can generate the **B cell coreceptor** ligand **C3d** (Figure 8–5).
   a. C3d can covalently bind to antigens.
   b. C3d–antigen complexes cross-link the BCR with **CR2,** which is composed of the CD19 and CD21 peptides.

c. Src kinases associated with CR2 promote BCR signaling through phosphorylation.

SWITCH RECOMBINASE DEFICIENCY

- *Ig class switching involves a DNA recombination event mediated by the recombinase **activation-induced cytidine deaminase (AID)**.*
- *Mutations in the AID gene have been described and result in impaired antigen-induced isotype switching, somatic hypermutation in B cells, and affinity maturation of the antibody response.*
- *The resulting phenotype, designated **hyper-IgM syndrome type 2**, resembles the X-linked CD154 deficiency known as **hyper-IgM syndrome type 1**.*

    F. Cytokines produced by T helper cells promote B cell activation.
      1. Interleukin (IL)-2, IL-4, and IL-5 promote B cell proliferation.
      2. IL-6 enhances the differentiation of activated B cells into antibody-producing plasma cells.
      3. IL-2, IL-4, and IL-6 promote antibody synthesis by activated B cells and plasma cells.
      4. Several cytokines promote Ig class switching.
        a. Switch cytokines promote specific **switch recombinase** interactions with specific switch sites within the Ig H gene locus (Chapter 4).
        b. IL-4 and IL-13 promote switching to IgE.
        c. Interferon (IFN)-γ promotes switching to IgG_1 and IgG_3.
        d. IL-5 and transforming growth factor-β (TGF-β) induce switching to IgA.

ANTICYTOKINE THERAPIES FOR CONTROLLING B CELL ACTIVATION

- *Monoclonal antibodies capable of neutralizing cytokines or blocking their receptors have potential for the treatment of allergic or neoplastic diseases involving B cells.*
- *For example, atopic allergies could theoretically be treated by blocking B cell switching to IgE synthesis with anti-IL-4 or anti-IL-13.*
- *Another application undergoing clinical trials is the use of anti-IL-6 or anti-IL-6 receptor antibodies to inhibit the growth and Ig production of myeloma cells.*

  IV. Foreign polysaccharides, glycolipids, and nucleic acids induce antibody production without the need for T cell help.
    A. These **T-independent (TI) antigens** contain repeating epitopes that cross-link multiple BCRs on a single B cell.
    B. Some TI antigens (eg, bacterial LPS) also coactivate B cells through Toll-like receptors (Chapter 1).
    C. Some TI antigens [eg, lipopolysaccharide (LPS)] can activate complement and coactivate B cells through CR2.
    D. Because TI antigens are not presented by antigen-presenting cells (APCs), they do not activate $CD4^+$ Th cells.
    E. The responses to TI antigens differ from responses to foreign proteins.
      1. There is little **Ig class switching** in TI antibody responses; IgM and IgG_2 antibodies predominate.
      2. A limited repertoire of antibody-mediated **effector functions** results.

3. **Memory B cell** populations are not formed and **affinity maturation** through somatic hypermutation does not occur.

4. **High-titered antibody** responses are not seen on secondary challenge.

SELECTIVE IGG₂ DEFICIENCY

- *IgG₂ is a common subclass of antibody produced in response to T-independent antigens in humans.*
- *Antibody responses to protein antigens are predominantly of the IgG₁ subclass.*
- *Children with selective IgG₂ subclass deficiency have difficulty clearing bacteria that express polysaccharide capsules (eg, Streptococcus pneumoniae and Haemophilus influenzae).*
- *The increased survival of encapsulated bacteria in IgG₂-deficient patients suggests that other (sub)classes of Igs do not provide sufficient host defense against these organisms.*

V. Antibody responses at mucosal surfaces are mediated by a specialized set of B cells that synthesizes IgA antibodies.

  A. Most of the IgA in the body is synthesized in the small intestine.

  B. IgA-secreting plasma cells are most abundant within the lamina propria of the submucosum and produce 2 g of Ig per day.

  C. The secretory form of IgA is the central mediator of mucosal humoral immunity.

    1. Secretory IgA is dimeric and contains J chain and **secretory component (SC)** (Chapter 3).

      a. The α, κ, λ, and J chains of dimeric IgA are produced by mucosal B cells.

      b. Secretory component is synthesized by the intestinal **epithelial cell**.

    2. Secretory component mediates transepithelial transport of IgA.

      a. On the basolateral surface of epithelial cells, a precursor of SC called **poly-Ig receptor** is expressed (Figure 9–3).

      b. The poly-Ig receptor binds the polymeric Igs (IgA and IgM).

      c. The loaded receptor is internalized into endosomes, which are translocated to the apical cell surface.

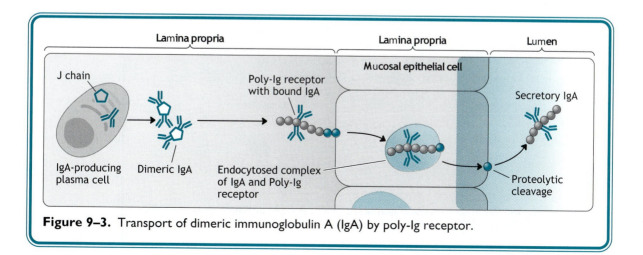

Figure 9–3. Transport of dimeric immunoglobulin A (IgA) by poly-Ig receptor.

d. Proteolytic cleavage of the poly-Ig receptor releases secretory component with its polymeric Ig attached.

D. At the mucosal surface, secretory IgA neutralizes toxins and allergens and prevents microbial entry.

SELECTIVE IGA DEFICIENCY

- *Selective IgA antibody deficiency is the most common antibody deficiency in humans with frequencies as high as 1:333 reported in some populations.*
- *This deficiency is characterized by recurrent bacterial and viral infections originating at mucosal surfaces (respiratory, gastrointestinal, and genitourinary tract infections).*
- *Increased incidences of food allergies, autoimmunity, and certain types of cancers have also been reported in these patients.*
- *However, half of all persons with this deficiency are asymptomatic.*

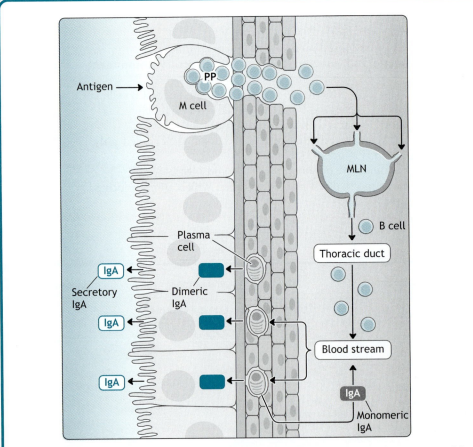

Figure 9–4. Induction of a mucosal immunoglobulin A (IgA) antibody response. M, microfold; PP, Peyer's patch; MLN, mesenteric lymph node.

- *The absence of increased rates of infection in the unaffected subset of IgA-deficient individuals probably reflects the translocation of secretory IgM by the poly-Ig receptor.*

   E. Mucosal IgA antibody responses are initially induced within submucosal Peyer's patches of the small intestine (Figure 9–4).
     1. The epithelium overlying the patch is composed of specialized nonvillous epithelial cells, called **M cells**, which efficiently transport antigens to lymphoid cells within the patch.
     2. Peyer's patch Th cells produce IL-5 and TGF-β, two IgA switch cytokines.
     3. B cells activated in the Peyer's patches migrate via draining lymph nodes into the lymph and blood.
     4. Circulating IgA-expressing B cells then seed the intestine and other **mucosal-associated lymphoid tissues (MALT)**.
     5. By this process, the recognition of enteric antigens leads to the production and transport of secretory IgA at multiple mucosal tissue sites.

MUCOSAL AND PARENTERAL VACCINES

- *In the 1950s two competing vaccines were produced against the polio virus.*
- *The parenteral (Salk) vaccine was injected by the intramuscular route and induced IgG antibody production.*
- *These antibodies prevented disease by neutralizing virus particles in transit from the gastrointestinal tract to the nervous tissues.*
- *The Sabin vaccine was an inactivated virus, and oral immunization resulted in secretory IgA responses in the gut-associated lymphoid tissues.*
- *Secretory IgA antibodies prevented viral attachment and entry into intestinal epithelial cells.*
- *Current recommendations are for children to receive the parenteral vaccine at 2, 4, and 6 months of age (www.cdc.gov/nip/recs/child-schedule.PDF).*

CLINICAL PROBLEMS

A patient is shown to have a mutation in his *Btk* tyrosine kinase gene.

1. Which of the following stages of lymphocyte differentiation is blocked in this patient?
   A. Differentiation of mature B cells into plasma cells
   B. Generation of memory B cells
   C. Differentiation of pre-B cells into immature B cells
   D. Negative selection of mature B cells
   E. Activation of mature B cells

A patient presents with recurrent bacterial infections and is found to have low serum levels of IgA and IgG$_1$, but elevated concentrations of serum IgM. Flow cytometry of his lymph node cells reveals an absence of CD154.

2. In which of the following areas of the lymph node would this cell surface marker normally be found?

A. Medullary cords

B. Diffuse cortex

C. Germinal centers

D. High endothelial cells of the venules

E. Subcapsular sinuses

Lymphocytes from an immunodeficient patient are found to lack mRNA for AID.

3. Which of the following lymphocyte subsets would be expected to be absent in this patient?

A. Lymph node B cells expressing membrane IgG

B. CD4$^+$ T lymphocytes in the blood

C. Natural killer (NK) cells in the spleen

D. All lymphocytes in peripheral lymphoid tissues

E. CD19$^+$ B cells in the bone marrow

You have a patient with recurrent infections, but normal T cell function.

4. Which of the following laboratory tests would help you determine if this immune deficiency is due to an *absence* of B cells?

A. Radioimmunoassay

B. Flow cytometry

C. Enzyme-linked immunosorbent assay (ELISA)

D. Immunofixation

E. Coombs test

A lymph node biopsy stained with hematoxylin and eosin shows numerous germinal centers in the superficial cortex.

5. Which of the following best describes the source of this biopsy tissue?

A. A patient who lacks CD154

B. A patient who lacks Rag1

C. A patient who has been immunized repeatedly with a protein vaccine

D. A patient who has been immunized repeatedly with streptococcal polysaccharides

E. A newborn

ANSWERS

1. The correct answer is C. Whereas the Btk kinase is used for both BCR and pre-BCR signaling, an absence of Btk is manifest first in pre-B cells. The mutation causes defective positive selection of pre-B cells and apoptotic death. There are no peripheral immature or mature B cells in Btk-deficient individuals, a condition known as XLA.

2. The correct answer is B. CD154 would normally be found on Th cells in the diffuse or deep cortex. Its absence is indicative of hyper-IgM syndrome type 1.

3. The correct answer is A. The switch recombinase AID is normally expressed in B cells that are undergoing Ig isotype switching.

4. The correct answer is B. Only flow cytometry would be able to demonstrate the absence of B cells. The other techniques would not distinguish between an absence of B cells and the inability of those cells to secrete antibody.

5. The correct answer is C. Germinal center development is antigen, Th cell, and CD40 dependent. The antigen must be a T-dependent antigen, such as a protein. Polysaccharide antigens do not induce germinal center formation, and newborns have generally not encountered protein antigens in utero that elicit this type of response.

CHAPTER 10
T CELL DIFFERENTIATION AND FUNCTION

I. The development of T lymphocytes is similar to that of B cells, although unique events occur in the inductive environment of the **thymus.**

   A. Thymic maturation does not require exposure to foreign antigen.

   B. Like B cells, T cells are derived from pluripotent **hematopoietic stem cells** in the fetal liver and bone marrow, which differentiate into common **lymphoid progenitor cells** and **progenitor T (pro-T) cells** (Table 10–1).

   C. The pro-T cell begins its migration from the bone marrow to the thymus during the first trimester of human pregnancy.

   D. In the thymus the cells are called **thymocytes** and undergo considerable cell division and apoptotic death.

      1. Differentiation is induced by **stromal cells** and **growth factors.**

         a. Epithelial cells, macrophages, and dendritic cells provide both contact-dependent and secreted signals.

         b. **Interleukin (IL)-7** is a key growth-promoting factor for thymocytes.

         c. Major histocompatibility complex (MHC) molecules promote thymocyte growth and apoptosis.

      2. Thymocytes are subjected to both positive and negative selection based on the specificity of their T cell receptors (TCRs).

   E. The production of mature T cells occurs throughout life, but the thymus becomes less important as it atrophies with age.

THE BUBBLE BOY

CLINICAL CORRELATION

- *In the 1976 movie "Boy in a Bubble," a child with a severe immunodeficiency avoided life-threatening infections by living in a pathogen-free plastic tent.*
- *A number of molecular defects can cause this condition, known as **severe combined immune deficiency**.*
- *These include mutations in the genes for the Rag recombinases, adenosine deaminase, and the γ chain of the IL-2 receptor (Chapter 16).*
- *The microbial pathogens that establish early opportunistic infections in these children include intracellular fungi, viruses, and bacteria.*
- *While B cell differentiation can also be directly or indirectly affected (depending on the mutation), maternal IgG provides immune protection early in life.*
- *Hematopoietic stem cell transplantation provides the only practical cure.*

Table 10–1. Stages of T cell differentiation.[a]

	HSC	Pro-T	Pre-T	Double Positive	Single Positive	Naive Mature T Cell
Rag	−	+	−	+	−	−
TdT	−	+	−	−	−	−
TCR DNA	Germline	Germline	Rearranged β chain	Rearranged β and α chain	Rearranged β and α chain	Rearranged β and α chain
TCR	None	None	Pre-TCR	TCR	TCR	TCR
CD3	−	−	+	+	+	+
Surface markers	−	−	−	CD4$^+$8$^+$	CD4$^+$ or CD8$^+$	CD4$^+$ or CD8$^+$
Anatomic site	Bone marrow	Thymus	Thymus	Thymus	Thymus	Periphery
Response to TCR ligation	None	None	Positive selection	Positive and negative selection	Negative selection	Activation

[a]Tdt, terminal deoxynucleotidyltransferase.

II. Thymocyte differentiation is accompanied by the generation of the TCR repertoire and the establishment of functional cell subsets.

A. Four important events in the development of the T cell lineage occur.
  1. TCRαβ and TCRγδ genes are rearranged by recombination (Chapter 6) and are expressed.
  2. The MHC restriction specificity of the T cell lineage is established.
  3. Thymocytes with autoreactive TCRs are eliminated.
  4. Two major functional T cell subsets (CD4$^+$ and CD8$^+$) are generated.

B. Clonal proliferation, apoptotic death, and differential gene expression accompany thymocyte differentiation.
  1. **Pro-T** cells migrate to the superficial cortex and become part of the pool of **double-negative (CD4$^-$CD8$^-$)** thymocytes (Table 10–1 and Table 10–2).
    a. Pro-T cells begin to express recombination activating genes 1 and 2 (Rag1, Rag2) and terminal deoxynucleotidyltransferase (TdT) in preparation for TCRβ locus rearrangements.
    b. In most pro-T cells, the β locus undergoes D–J rearrangement.
    c. Approximately 5% of the descendants of these cells will express γδ TCRs and the remainder will become TCRαβ$^+$.
  2. Pro-T cells then differentiate into **pre-T cells**, in which V–DJ$_\beta$ joining occurs and a β chain polypeptide is expressed.

Table 10–2. The major subsets of the TCRαβ lineage of thymocytes.[a]

Thymocyte Subset	Surface Phenotype	Major Events or Properties
Double negative		
Pro-T cell	$CD4^-CD8^-TCR^-$	$TdT^+Rag1,2^+$; $D\text{-}J_\beta$ rearrangement
Pre-T cell	$CD4^-CD8^-TCR^-CD3^+pre\text{-}TCR^+$	$Rag1,2^+$; $V\text{-}DJ_\beta$ rearrangement
Double positive	$CD4^+CD8^+CD3^+TCR\alpha\beta^+$	$V\text{-}J_\alpha$ rearrangement
		Positive and negative selection
Single positive		
$CD4^+$	$CD4^+CD8^-CD3^+TCR\alpha\beta^+$	Negative selection
$CD8^+$	$CD4^-CD8^+CD3^+TCR\alpha\beta^+$	Negative selection

[a]TCR, T cell receptor.

    a. A **pre-TCR** is expressed that contains a β chain plus a **pre-Tα chain** and CD3 peptides.
    b. Activation of pre-T cells through the pre-TCR stimulates cell proliferation, β locus allelic exclusion, α locus rearrangement, and the expression of CD4 and CD8.
  3. Double positive thymocytes express TCRαβ with CD3 peptides.
    a. Rag1,2 are expressed for a second time to facilitate rearrangement of the α locus.
    b. TCRαβ binding to MHC molecules signals further maturation.
      (1) Rag1,2 genes become silent.
      (2) Positive and negative selection occurs as the cells transition to a single positive ($CD4^+8^-$ or $CD4^-8^+$) state.
  4. Single positive cells emerge from the thymus and undergo further maturation in the peripheral lymphoid tissues.
  5. The maturation of thymocytes can be monitored by polychromatic flow cytometry (Figure 10–1).
    a. Using antibodies to CD4 and CD8, each with a different fluorochrome, four cell subsets can be identified.
      (1) Double negative ($CD4^-CD8^-$) cells are the pro-T and pre-T cells.
      (2) Double positive ($CD4^+CD8^+$) cells express TCRαβ or TCRγδ and are positively and negatively selected based on their TCR specificities.
      (3) Single positive ($CD4^+CD8^-$ or $CD4^-CD8^+$) cells are fairly mature and ready to exit the thymus.
    b. A similar analysis of peripheral T cells would identify only the two single-positive subsets.

SIGNIFICANCE OF ORAL THRUSH IN INFANTS

• *A cardinal clinical sign of defective cellular immunity in a neonate is the appearance of mucocutaneous candidiasis or **thrush**.*

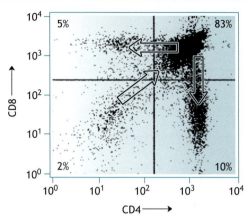

Figure 10–1. Identification of the major subsets of thymocytes by flow cytometry. (Courtesy of Thomas Yankee, University of Kansas Medical Center)

- *Oral thrush is uncommon in immunocompetent individuals.*
- *This painful condition is caused by a superficial infection by the opportunistic yeast* Candida albicans, *which is normal flora in the oral cavity.*
- *The most frequent immune deficiency causing neonatal thrush is AIDS.*
- *However, any cellular immune deficiency, including severe combined immunodeficiency (SCID), selective T cell deficiencies (eg, DiGeorge syndrome, CD3 mutations), and MHC deficiencies, can increase the risk of thrush.*

III. Host MHC molecules determine the specificities of the TCRs that survive thymic selection.

A. The **potential repertoire** of TCRαβ and TCRγδ receptors is determined by the quasirandom recombination events within the DNA that codes for TCR V regions (Chapter 6).

B. The **utilized repertoire** of TCRs results from the selection of receptors with the ability to recognize foreign peptides presented by the MHC of the host.

C. The affinity with which thymocyte TCRs bind MHC molecules in the thymus determines whether positive or negative selection will occur.
  1. In the absence of binding, thymocytes undergo death by neglect.
  2. Low-affinity TCR–MHC interactions trigger positive selection.
  3. High-affinity TCR binding to MHC signals negative selection.

D. Positive selection promotes the development of thymocytes with TCRs specific for foreign peptides plus the host's own MHC molecules.
  1. Cells bearing TCRs specific for non-self MHC (ie, that of another individual) die by neglect.
  2. **Positive selection** occurs at the double-positive thymocyte stage and induces differentiation to the single-positive phenotype.
     a. Double-positive thymocytes with TCRs that bind to self MHC *class I* molecules are induced to become CD4⁻CD8⁺.

b. Double positive thymocytes with TCRs that bind to MHC *class II* molecules become CD4$^+$CD8$^-$ single positive.

    c. Clones that express TCRs specific for nonhost MHC class I or II are not positively selected and die by default.

    d. The majority of developing thymocytes are *not* positively selected and undergo apoptosis.

MHC DEFICIENCIES PREVENT POSITIVE SELECTION

- *Two important groups of immune deficiency diseases result from inefficient positive selection of thymocytes.*
- ***Bare lymphocyte syndrome (BLS)*** *type 1 and type 2 (Chapter 7) are congenital deficiencies in which MHC class I and class II molecules, respectively, are not expressed.*
- *The absence of MHC molecules precludes positive selection of double positive thymocytes and the corresponding T cell subset fails to develop.*
- *For example, BLS type 2 patients are lymphopenic, because CD4$^+$ T cells, which normally constitute the majority of T cells in the blood, do not develop.*
- *The differential diagnosis of BLS type 2 requires exclusion of HIV-1 infection, which is a much more common cause of decreased CD4:CD8 ratios (Chapter 15).*

    E. Negative selection eliminates potentially harmful thymocyte clones that bear high affinity receptors for self peptides plus self MHC molecules.

      1. Negative selection establishes **central tolerance** to self antigens (Chapter 16).

      2. Negative selection occurs at the double positive-to-single positive transition.

      3. Both MHC class I and class II can signal negative selection.

      4. Coreceptor signaling through CD4 and CD8 promotes negative selection.

      5. The death signal during negative selection is delivered through **Fas–Fas ligand** interactions between thymocytes and stromal cells of the thymus.

    F. Four potential outcomes result from the binding of peptide–MHC complexes by TCRs.

      1. Thymocyte clones are induced to proliferate and differentiate (positive selection).

      2. Thymocyte clones undergo apoptosis (negative selection).

      3. Peripheral T cells proliferate and differentiate in response to foreign antigens.

      4. Peripheral T cells can become anergic (**peripheral tolerance**) if coreceptor signaling is lacking (Chapter 16).

DEFECTIVE THYMIC APOPTOSIS

- *Apoptotic death regulates thymocyte selection and T cell activation in the periphery.*
- ***Autoimmune lymphoproliferative syndrome (ALPS)*** *(also known as Canale–Smith syndrome) is a defect in the apoptosis of activated T cells.*
- *In most patients a mutation exists in the gene coding for **Fas** (CD95).*
- *Patients present with greatly enlarged lymph nodes, splenomegaly, and autoimmunity (eg, Coombs-positive hemolytic anemias).*
- *Affected individuals also show lymphocytosis and an elevated number of double negative (TCRαβ$^+$CD4$^-$CD8$^-$) T cells in the blood.*
- *Similar phenotypes occur with patients bearing mutations in Fas ligand or certain caspase genes.*

IV. Cell surface **adhesion molecules, coreceptors, and cytokine receptors** regulate T cell activation in the periphery.

A. **Cell adhesion molecules** promote T cell homing to specific tissues by binding to ligands on vascular endothelial cells and matrix proteins.

1. T cells express **integrins**, such as **lymphocyte function-associated antigen-1 (LFA-1)**, that mediate lymphocyte homing to sites of infection and inflammation.

2. Specialized integrins direct T cells to mucosal lymphoid tissues.

3. Integrins increase the avidity of binding between T cells and their antigen-presenting cells.

4. Integrins promote binding between cytotoxic T cells and their target cells.

B. **Coreceptors** are induced and recruited to the **immunological synapse** that forms between a T cell and its antigen-presenting cell.

1. The cell surface expression of coreceptors and their ligands is often regulated to avoid the unwanted activation of resting T cells.

2. Receptor clustering brings coreceptors in proximity to TCRs.

3. Receptor clustering promotes synergy between intracellular signaling pathways.

4. **CD4** and **CD8** are coreceptors that bind to nonpolymorphic residues of MHC class II and class I molecules, respectively.

    a. The T cell-specific kinase **Lck** is associated with CD4 and CD8 in the membrane.

    b. Lck phosphorylates immunotyrosine activation motif (ITAM) residues on CD3 peptides.

    c. Thymocytes lacking Lck are not positively selected at the double-positive stage.

5. **CD28** and **cytotoxic T lymphocyte-associated protein 4 (CTLA-4)** (CD152) on T cells modify TCR signaling.

    a. The **costimulatory ligands** for these coreceptors are members of the B7 family and are expressed on antigen-presenting cells.

    b. Ligation of CD28 on naive T cells by B7 induces phosphatidylinositol-3-kinase activation.

    c. Stimulation of T cells through CD28 activates NFκB.

    d. CTLA-4 is expressed on activated T cells and mediates negative signaling when B7 is bound.

6. **CD154** is a coreceptor for CD4$^+$ Th cells.

C. **Cytokine receptors** augment or inhibit T cell responses to antigen.

1. The expression of cytokine receptors is often induced by antigen and coreceptor stimulation.

2. **IL-2** is a growth factor for activated CD4$^+$ and CD8$^+$ T cells.

3. **IL-4** promotes the differentiation of the Th2 subset from naive, antigen-stimulated CD4$^+$ T cells.

4. **Interferon (IFN)-γ** promotes the differentiation of the Th1 subset of T cells.

5. **IL-10** and **transforming growth factor (TGF-β)** inhibit the activation of Th1 cells.

6. **IFN-γ** inhibits the activation of Th2 cells.

D. Different types of costimulatory and cytokine signals are derived from different types of antigen-presenting cells (Table 10–3).

Table 10–3. Differences between APCs related to T cell activation.[a]

Property	Dendritic Cell	B Cell	Macrophage
Antigen uptake	Active endocytosis	BCR-mediated endocytosis	Endocytosis and phagocytosis
MHC class II expression	Constitutive	Constitutive	Inducible
Costimulatory ligand expression	Constitutive B7	Inducible B7	Inducible B7
T cells activated	Naive, effector and memory	Effector and memory	Effector and memory

[a]APC, antigen-presenting cells; BCR, B cell receptor.

1. **Dendritic cells** are particularly effective at activating naive CD4$^+$ T cells, because they express B7 and MHC class II constitutively.
2. **B cells** have the advantage of being able to capture limited quantities of antigen through their BCR, which aids in activating memory T cells with high-affinity TCRs.
3. **Macrophages** can phagocytize particulate antigens and present their epitopes to T cells.

V. **The activation of mature T cells by antigen in the periphery leads to clonal expansion and differentiation into effector and memory cell subsets.**
   A. The frequency of T cells specific for a given antigen changes during an immune response.
      1. Clonal frequencies among resting naive T cells is approximately 10^{-6}.
      2. The frequency of antigen-specific T cells increases to 10^{-2} at the peak of the expansion phase.
      3. Memory cells for a given antigen exist at a frequency of 10^{-4}.
   B. CD4$^+$ helper T cells (Th cells) can be subdivided into two subsets (Figure 6–5).
      1. **Th1 cells** mediate cellular immunity to intracellular microbial pathogens by the secretion of cytokines [eg, IL-2, IFN-γ, and tumor necrosis factor (TNF)-α] that promote T cell growth and activate macrophages and neutrophils.
      2. **Th2 cells** promote humoral immunity to extracellular microbial pathogens by producing cytokines (IL-4, IL-5, and IL-13) that activate B cells.
   C. **Memory T cells** divide at a low rate and recirculate for decades.
      1. The chemokine receptor CCR7 and certain adhesion molecules facilitate memory T cell migration into lymph nodes.
      2. The antigen-presenting cell (APC) signals required to activate a memory T cell with antigen are different than those required by naive T cells (Table 10–2).
      3. Memory T cells become a greater proportion of the T cell pool with age.

D. Regulatory T (Treg) cells inhibit immune responses (Chapter 11).
   1. Treg cells are most often CD4⁺ and express **CD25**, the α chain of the high-affinity IL-2 receptor.
   2. Treg cells produce the inhibitory cytokines **IL-10** and **TGF-β**.
   3. Treg cells contribute to the maintenance of self tolerance (Chapter 16).

E. Several subsets of T cells and related lymphocytes are **cytotoxic** (Table 10–4).
   1. Cytotoxic T lymphocytes (CTL) are induced by antigen, terminally differentiated and short lived.
      a. Most CTL are CD8⁺ and MHC class I restricted.
      b. Cytotoxic CD4⁺ cells exist, but are MHC class II restricted.
      c. Both TCRαβ and TCRγδ T cells can be cytotoxic.
      d. Cytotoxicity is mediated by the granzyme–perforin pathway, the Fas–Fas ligand pathway, and the TNF receptor pathway (Chapter 6).
   2. The **γδ T cell** subset shows specificity for pathogens associated with epithelial surfaces.
      a. γδ T cells are **intraepithelial lymphocytes** that accumulate in the skin, small intestine, lung, and genitourinary tract.
      b. Most TCRγδ⁺ cells do not express CD4 or CD8.
      c. TCRγδ is specific for nonpeptides, including glycolipids that represent pathogen-associated molecular patterns.
      d. TCRγδ is not MHC restricted.

Table 10–4. A comparison of conventional T cells, γδ T cells, NKT cells, and NK cells.[a]

Property	Conventional T Cell	γδ T Cell	NKT Cell	NK Cell
Tissue location	Spleen, lymph nodes, lymphoid follicles	Intraepithelial	Thymus, liver, spleen	Liver > spleen
Receptor type	TCRαβ + CD3	TCRγδ + CD3	Invariant TCRαβ + CD3	Activating FcγR NKG2D Inhibitory KIR Lectins
Receptor specificity	Peptide + MHC class I or class II	Microbial glycolipids	Microbial glycolipids Stress-induced host ligands There are two receptor types and two receptor specificities: activating and inhibitory	Activating IgG antibody Stress-induced host ligands Inhibitory HLA-A,B,C

[a]NKT, natural killer T; TCR, T cell receptor; MHC, major histocompatibility complex; KIR, killer inhibitory receptor; IgG, immunoglobulin G.

e. Signaling through **TCRγδ** is similar to that of TCRαβ.
   f. γδ T cells can be cytotoxic or cytokine producing.
3. **Natural killer T (NKT) cells** express both TCRs and NK cell markers.
   a. The invariant TCRαβ of NKT cells is restricted by CD1 and specific for microbial glycolipids.
   b. NKT cells respond rapidly to antigen and produce IL-4 and IFN-γ.
F. Although not thymus derived, **NK cells** share a number of properties with T cells and NKT cells.
   1. NK cells recognize host cells infected with intracellular microbial pathogens using unique receptors.
      a. NK cell **inhibitory receptors** recognize MHC class I molecules and deliver signals that are dominant over NK cell-**activating receptor** signals.
      b. NK cell-**activating receptors** recognize host cell ligands that are present on infected or stressed cells.
      c. When host cells fail to express MHC class I (as during virus infections), the inhibitory signal is lost and the NK cell becomes activated.
      d. Activating receptors signal through their ITAMs and inhibitory receptors utilize **immunotyrosine *inhibitory*** motifs (ITIMs) to transmit intracellular signals.
      e. The functions of NK cells are promoted by cytokines.
   2. NK cells mediate innate immunity by producing cytokines (eg, IFN-γ) and killing infected target cells without the need for clonal expansion.
   3. Important coactivating signals for NK cells include IL-12 and IFN-α/β.

CHEDIAK–HIGASHI SYNDROME

- *Chediak–Higashi Syndrome (CHS) is a rare autosomal recessive condition characterized by recurrent infections and poor NK cell activity.*
- *The genetic defect resides in the gene for **lysosomal trafficking regulator (LYST)** and causes a fusion of cytoplasmic granules in NK cells, neutrophils, monocytes, and other granule-containing cells.*
- *CHS NK cells bind normally to their target cells, but killing is absent.*
- *The immune deficiencies of CHS patients are probably more related to defective neutrophil function than impaired NK cell activity.*

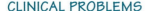

CLINICAL PROBLEMS

You have a patient with enlarged lymph nodes, splenomegaly, and anemia. During an immunological work-up you find that the patient has a slight lymphocytosis. You perform multicolor flow cytometry after staining the patient's blood lymphocytes with antibodies to CD3, CD4, and CD8. Shown below are CD3⁺ blood lymphocytes stained for CD4 (x-axis) and CD8 (y-axis) expression.

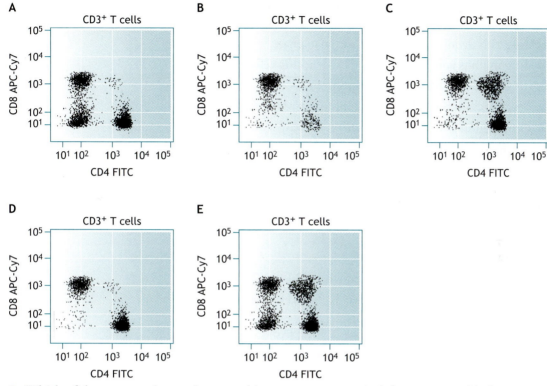

1. Which of the patterns shown above would suggest an apoptosis defect is responsible for this patient's disease?

   A. A

   B. B

   C. C

   D. D

   E. E

A patient with BLS type 1 presents with a herpes virus infection. His blood lymphocytes are found to kill autologous virus-infected target cells rapidly in vitro.

2. Which of the following cell types is probably mediating this killing?

   A. CD8⁺ T cells

   B. γδ T cells

   C. Macrophages

   D. NK cells

   E. B cells

You are a member of a cardiac transplantation team in a medical school and meet with second-year medical students to explain the surgical procedure and posttransplantation therapy. One of the drugs you review is cyclosporine.

3. Which of the following would be a reasonable summary of its immunosuppressive effect?

A. The drug kills dividing T and B cells in metaphase.

B. The drug inhibits antigen processing by dendritic cells.

C. The drug inhibits IL-2 gene transcription in T cells.

D. The drug blocks NK cell recognition of foreign HLA antigens.

E. The drug inhibits HLA class I expression by cardiac muscle cells.

Mutations in either Rag1 or Rag2 cause severe immunodeficiencies in human beings.

4. Which of the following cell types would show normal numbers in a patient with a Rag1 deficiency?

A. CD3⁺ cells with a CD4 coreceptor

B. CD19⁺ cells

C. Single positive thymocytes

D. Lymphocytes with a coreceptor specific for C3d

E. Cells with an inhibitory receptor specific for MHC class I

Johnny is an 8-month-old child with recurrent viral and fungal infections. His blood lymphocytes can bind IL-2, and his macrophages can bind IFN-γ in vitro. It has been determined that his parents are both heterozygous for a mutation in the ZAP-70 gene known to disrupt the activity of this kinase.

5. Assuming Johnny has inherited this mutation from both parents, which of his cells should be *normal*?

A. Monocytes and macrophages

B. TCRαβ T lymphocytes

C. TCRγδ T lymphocytes

D. NK cells

E. NKT cells

ANSWERS

1. The correct answer is A. This pattern is abnormal in the sense that the blood contains large numbers of double negative T lymphocytes (CD3⁺CD4⁻CD8⁻). Normally, double negative CD3⁺ cells are found only in the thymus (panel E). This finding suggests altered thymic selection and peripheral homeostasis of T cell subsets secondary to defective apoptosis induced by the Fas–Fas ligand system (ie, autoimmune lymphoproliferative syndrome). The normal pattern for blood CD3⁺ cells is shown in panel D.

2. The correct answer is D. NK cells recognize virus-infected and neoplastic cells that lack MHC class I, which is characteristic of cells from patients with BLS type 1.

3. The correct answer is C. Cyclosporine inhibits the Ca^{2+}/calmodulin-dependent phosphatase calcineurin, which leads to decreased TCR-initiated dephosphorylation of the latent transcription factor NFAT. With diminished NFAT activation, IL-2 and IL-4 gene transcription is decreased, which has a general immunosuppressive effect on activated T cells.

4. The correct answer is E. $T^-B^-NK^+$ SCID is caused by Rag recombinase deficiency. The patients have normal numbers of NK cells, which bear inhibitory receptors for MHC class I molecules.

5. The correct answer is A. All of the lymphocyte subsets listed use ZAP-70 as a signaling intermediate for receptor-induced cell activation.

CHAPTER 11
REGULATION OF IMMUNE RESPONSES

I. The immune response is regulated at the level of antigen recognition by mechanisms designed to distinguish self from nonself.

    A. The innate immune system recognizes **pathogen-associated molecular patterns** that are not seen on host tissues.

    B. The adaptive immune system recognizes nonself **epitopes** using T and B cell receptor repertoires that have been selected for their specificity during lymphocyte differentiation.

    C. Both systems are imperfect, and immune responses to self components can arise even in healthy individuals (Chapter 16).

        1. Toll-like receptors recognize self components derived from damaged tissues (eg, heat shock proteins).

        2. Antibody production against self antigens occurs frequently without any adverse effect.

II. Antigen-presenting cells (APCs) control the induction of adaptive immune responses.

    A. The constellation of major histocompatibility complex (MHC) molecules expressed by an APC determines the peptides it can present.

    B. **Coreceptor signals** derived from APCs influence the type of immune response induced.

        1. Whereas mature dendritic cells (DC) activate CD4$^+$ Th cells, immature DC activate CD4$^+$ Treg cells.

        2. CD28 binding of B7 molecules induces Th cell activation, whereas cytotoxic T lymphocyte-associated protein 4 (CTLA-4) binding of B7 molecules inhibits Th cell activation.

    C. **Cytokines** influence APC functions and lymphocyte activation.

        1. Interferon (IFN)-γ and tumor necrosis factor (TNF)-α increase MHC class II expression and APC function.

        2. Macrophage- and DC-derived interleukin (IL)-12 promotes Th1 cell activation.

        3. IL-4 produced by T cells and mast cells promotes Th2 cell differentiation.

III. When an immune response does occur, its duration is limited, and the immune system returns to a basal homeostatic state.

    A. As antigen is cleared from the body, lymphocyte activation subsides.

B. Antigen-activated lymphocytes undergo **activation-induced cell death**.

    1. Activated T lymphocytes express both **Fas** and **Fas ligand**, which signals apoptotic death.

        a. The cytoplamic domains of Fas contain death domains that bind adapter proteins, recruit and activate caspases, and trigger apoptosis.

        b. Fas deficiency in humans causes **autoimmune lymphoproliferative syndrome (ALPS)** (Chapter 10), the failure of activated T cells to undergo apoptosis.

    2. Oxidant production by activated cells initiates cell death through the endogenous apoptosis pathway.

C. Effector lymphocytes, neutrophils, and macrophages are relatively **short lived**.

D. Memory B and T cells show only **low levels of proliferation**.

E. **Antibodies** regulate immune responses to their antigens.

    1. Maternal antibodies that cross the placenta can interfere with the immunization of the newborn in the first few months of life.

    2. Complement-activating antibodies enhance B cell activation through the **CR2 coreceptor** (Chapter 9).

    3. Immune complexes containing immunoglobulin G (IgG) can also inhibit B cell activation (Figure 11–1).

        a. IgG antibody–antigen complexes can simultaneously bind to the **Fcγ receptor IIB (FcγRIIB)** and BCR.

        b. BCR cross-linking to FcγRIIB blocks B cell receptor (BCR) signaling.

            (1) The cytoplasmic tail of FcγRIIB contains **immunotyrosine inhibitory motifs (ITIMs)**, which recruit **Src homology 2 domain-containing inositol polyphosphate 5-phosphatase (SHIP)**.

            (2) SHIP disrupts phospholipase Cγ (PLCγ) and Bruton's tyrosine kinase (Btk) activation.

RHOGAM THERAPY

CLINICAL
CORRELATION

- *Hemolytic disease of the newborn (erythroblastosis fetalis) is caused when an Rh-negative mother produces IgG antibodies to the Rh antigens of her fetus.*
- *Fetal anemia and jaundice occur when these antibodies cross the placenta.*
- *To prevent this condition, Rh-negative mothers are given* **Rhogam** *(Rh-specific γ-globulin) during and immediately after pregnancy.*
- *Rhogam prevents immunization of the mother by clearing fetal erythrocytes from her blood circulation.*
- *Rhogam also cross-links the BCR and FcγRIIB on maternal B cells and inhibits maternal B cell activation.*

    4. IgG immune complex binding to macrophage **FcγRI** (CD64) also induces the release of **IL-10, transforming growth factor (TGF)-β**, and **prostaglandin E₂ (PGE₂),** all of which inhibit lymphocyte activation.

    5. Antibodies produced against the idiotypic determinants of a BCR can inhibit B cell activation.

        a. Autoantibodies against idiotypes are produced regularly during adaptive immune responses.

        b. Antiidiotype antibodies can block B cell activation by cross-linking the BCR to FcγRIIB.

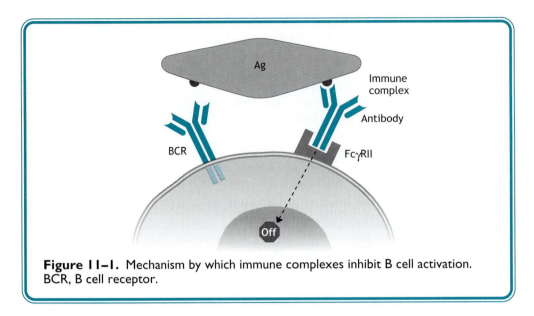

Figure 11–1. Mechanism by which immune complexes inhibit B cell activation. BCR, B cell receptor.

6. When high circulating antibody concentrations are achieved, the rate of Ig catabolism also increases.

INTRAVENOUS IMMUNOGLOBULIN (IVIG) THERAPY IN MULTIPLE MYELOMA

- *Multiple myeloma is characterized by pancytopenia due to the depression of hematopoiesis by the malignant cells within the bone marrow.*
- *This causes a functional **hypogammaglobulinemia** (ie, decreased production of useful antibodies) and increases the risk of infections.*
- *Prophylactic treatment with IVIG has not always proven useful for correcting this defect.*
- *The extremely high circulating levels of the M component cause an elevated clearance rate for all Ig, which limits the lifespan of exogenous IVIG.*

IV. CD4⁺CD25⁺ regulatory T cells (Treg cells) mediate immune homeostasis.

A. Treg cells suppress immune responses by several mechanisms.
   1. They consume IL-2 and deprive other lymphocytes of its growth-promoting activity.
   2. Treg cells inhibit activated T cells by cell–cell contact and the secretion of the inhibitory cytokines **IL-10** and **TGF-β**.
   3. Treg cells are induced late in immune responses and act by suppressing T cell effector functions.

B. Treg cells prevent immune-mediated diseases.
   1. Treg cells limit host tissue damage that might otherwise occur during exuberant immune responses to microbes.
   2. Treg cells assist in the maintenance of self tolerance and prevent autoimmunity.

THE IMMUNOLOGICAL ENIGMA OF PREGNANCY

- *In human pregnancies, the fetus is generally considered a* **semiallograft** *(ie, half of its tissue antigens are genetically foreign to the mother) (Chapter 17).*
- *It is not clear why such a foreign tissue graft is not rejected by the mother, but several mechanisms appear to contribute to fetal survival.*
- *Trophoblastic cells that form the fetal interface with the maternal circulation are devoid of most HLA antigens and certain costimulatory molecules, such as B7.*
- *Inhibitory factors, including IL-10, B7 isoforms, death receptor ligands, and PGE_2, are expressed at high levels at sites of implantation.*
- *Some fetal cells do cross the placenta and are tolerated by the mother's immune system for years after pregnancy, suggesting a central immune anergy.*

V. Polymorphisms exist in genes that regulate immune functions.

A. Dozens of genes that control immune cell differentiation and activation have been described, some of which will be discussed in Chapter 16.

    1. The majority of heritable defects in adaptive immunity have been genetically mapped, and the gene products have been identified.

    2. Much less is known about human genetic polymorphisms or mutations linked to defects in innate immunity.

B. Functionally significant mutations and polymorphisms in genes affecting complement components, components of antigen presentation pathways, cytokines, cytokine receptors, and Ig switch recombinases have been described.

VI. Dysregulation of the immune system can cause immunological diseases.

A. **Autoimmunity** occurs when self-tolerance is lost (Chapter 16).

    1. T cells specific for autoantigens can be activated when coreceptor ligands (eg, B7) are abnormally expressed.

    2. B cells that produce high affinity autoantibodies can be activated by costimulatory signals derived from infection.

    3. Defects in apoptosis (eg, Fas mutations) can result in a failure to delete autoreactive T cells.

B. Adaptive immune responses to microbial antigens can **cross-react** with self tissue antigens and cause immune-mediated tissue damage.

RHEUMATIC FEVER

- *Rheumatic fever in school age children is a complication secondary to pharyngitis caused by the bacterium Streptococcus pyogenes.*
- *Damage to the heart and joints appears 2–4 weeks after the pharyngitis.*
- *Antibodies produced against the streptococcal M protein* **cross-react** *with cardiac autoantigens.*
- *Autoantibodies to myosin, keratin, and laminin play a key role in cardiac valve damage.*

    C. **Atopic allergies** result when excessive immune responses are made to relatively innocuous environmental antigens (Chapter 13).

        1. Immune dysregulation causes **Th2 polarization.**

        2. IgE antibody production favors acute inflammatory responses.

    D. **Immune responses to microbes** can exceed what is necessary to clear the pathogen.

1. **Inflammatory bowel disease** results from immune responses to microbial flora that initiate chronic inflammation.
2. **Infectious mononucleosis** is caused by an excessive CD8+ T cell response to Epstein–Barr virus antigens that damages host tissues.

SEPSIS REVISITED

CLINICAL CORRELATION

- **Sepsis** *is a systemic inflammatory response to infection and one of the leading causes of death among hospitalized patients.*
- *The disease also illustrates what happens when immune mechanisms designed to protect the host are excessively activated (Figure 11–2).*
- *A complex pathogenesis results from the activation of multiple host defense systems by pathogenic and opportunistic microbes.*
- *Bacterial components, including lipopolysaccharide (LPS), can activate the complement, coagulation, and fibrinolysis systems.*
- *Macrophage activation for the production of proinflammatory cytokines (eg, TNF-α) and arachidonic acid metabolites results from Toll-like receptor stimulation.*
- *Endothelial and smooth muscle cells are activated, resulting in coagulopathies, severe hypotension, impaired organ perfusion, and hypoxic tissue damage.*

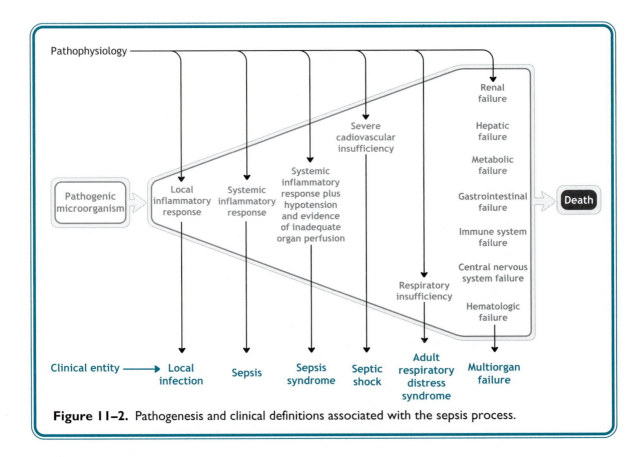

Figure 11–2. Pathogenesis and clinical definitions associated with the sepsis process.

CLINICAL PROBLEMS

Clinical vaccine trials using a nine-amino acid peptide immunogen from an HIV-1 glycoprotein have been performed. The vaccine is effective at inducing high-affinity IgG virus-neutralizing antibodies in only a subset of healthy adult vaccinees.

1. Which of the following immune properties probably characterizes the responsive individuals?

   A. They share HLA class II genes.

   B. They lack Treg cells.

   C. They are high producers of IL-10.

   D. They lack IL-2 receptors.

   E. They are all over 70 years of age.

A patient with lupus presents with impaired renal function, and a biopsy shows IgG and C3b deposits in the renal glomerulus. The patient's serum contains antibodies to her DNA and erythrocytes. Her total IgG is significantly elevated (1900 mg/dL).

2. Which of the following best explains the hypergammaglobulinemia seen in this patient?

   A. Reduced clearance of IgG by the damaged kidney

   B. Destruction of Treg cells by anti-DNA antibodies

   C. Polyclonal B cell activation by numerous self antigens

   D. An opportunistic virus infection

   E. Depletion of serum complement

Mary is a 2-year-old child with an unremarkable medical history, but presents today with enlarged cervical lymph nodes. Her complete blood count shows lymphocytosis (10,500/μL) and her serum contains elevated concentrations of IgG and IgM. Flow cytometry indicates that her CD3+ lymphocytes are 25% CD4+ and 20% CD8+. She has no history of recurrent infections and no evidence of a current infection or cancer.

3. Which of the following is the most likely basis for Mary's immune abnormalities?

   A. HIV-1 infection

   B. IgA deficiency

   C. Thymic hypoplasia (DiGeorge syndrome)

   D. An apoptosis defect (Fas deficiency)

   E. A monoclonal gammopathy

A 2-month-old healthy child is immunized with a new bacterial protein vaccine as part of a clinical trial. His preimmunization titer of IgG antibody to the vaccine protein is 1:16, and the titer is unchanged 2 weeks postimmunization.

4. Which of the following is a likely explanation for this observation?

A. The child has had an infection with the bacterium during gestation.

B. Maternal antibody to the bacterial protein blocked active immunization of the child.

C. The child has severe combined immune deficiency.

D. The child has a Th cell defect that prevents Ig class switching.

E. Children cannot make antibodies at this age.

ANSWERS

1. The correct answer is A. The high responding vacinees probably share HLA antigens that can present the peptide vaccine. Because this is an exogenous antigen, class II molecules would be involved. Presumably, the HLA class II molecules of the nonresponders failed to bind and present the peptide.

2. The correct answer is C. Elevated IgG levels in this patient are probably due to polyclonal B cell activation by autoantigens. Most patients of this type produce autoantibodies to a wide range of self antigens, suggesting that they have defects in general immune regulation mechanisms.

3. The correct answer is D. Mary has an unusual pattern of T cell markers. Only 45% of her T cells express either CD4 or CD8; the remaining T cells are apparently double negative. This is a classic sign of ALPS (Chapter 10). The condition arises from a defect in apoptosis among T cells resulting from a Fas mutation. Her elevated immunoglobulins probably represent autoantibodies against a range of self antigens, because self-reactive T cells are not controlled by Fas-mediated apoptosis.

4. The correct answer is B. The IgG antibodies present prior to immunization were probably maternally derived, because children of this age do not synthesize much IgG. The fact that the titer did not increase following immunization seems to indicate that the maternal antibodies interfered with B cell activation. This would occur if the vaccine and preformed maternal antibodies formed immunosuppressive immune complexes and cross-linked the BCR and FcγRIIB.

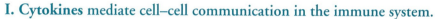

CHAPTER 12
CYTOKINES

I. Cytokines mediate cell–cell communication in the immune system.

    A. Cytokines are 8- to 25-kDa polypeptides that include **interleukins (IL),
chemokines, growth factors (GF), interferons (IFN)**, and **colony-stimulating
factors (CSF)** (Appendix II).

    B. Most cytokines are designed for rapid, short-term effects.

        1. They are often secreted immediately after their synthesis.

        2. Their short half-lives in circulation reflect the action of inactivators and bind-
ing proteins.

    C. Cytokines typically act over short distances.

        1. Many cytokines (eg, IL-2) have **autocrine** effects; they act on the cells that pro-
duce them.

        2. Other cytokines have localized **paracrine** effects; one cell produces a cytokine
that acts on a nearby cell.

        3. Cell–cell contact promotes the action of cytokines.

        4. A few cytokines show **endocrine** effects; they act at a distance after secretion
into the blood stream.

            a. Tumor necrosis factor (TNF)-α produced by tissue macrophages during
bacterial infections can have systemic inflammatory effects.

            b. IL-1β produced during inflammation or infections causes fever by its en-
docrine effects on the hypothalamus.

    D. Cytokines activate cells through specific high-affinity receptors.

        1. Dissociation constants for cytokine receptors are in the picomolar range.

        2. Receptors for cytokines that mediate acute inflammatory or innate immune re-
sponses are typically constitutively expressed.

        3. Receptors for lymphocyte-activating cytokines are often induced.

        4. The same receptor for a given cytokine may have significantly different effects
when expressed on different cell types.

    E. The most common cellular response to a cytokine is the rapid initiation of gene
transcription.

    F. Cytokines have **redundant** biological effects (Table 12–1).

        1. This ensures that a deficiency of one cytokine does not eliminate an essential
biological function.

        2. Cytokine redundancy frustrates anticytokine therapies.

    G. Most cytokines are **pleiotropic**; they exhibit several functions.

Table 12–1. Redundancies between TNF-α and IL-1β.[a]

Response	TNF-α	IL-1β
Fever induction	+	+
Acute phase protein induction through IL-6	+	+
Induction of vascular adhesion molecule expression	+	+
Induction of IL-8	+	+
Activation of NFκB	+	+
Joint inflammation in rheumatoid arthritis	+	+
Systemic inflammatory response syndrome (SIRS)	+	+
Cachexia	+	–
Induction of apoptosis	+	–

[a]TNF, tumor necrosis factor; IL, interleukin.

H. When combined, cytokines can have **synergistic** effects.
   1. One cytokine may induce the expression of receptors for the second cytokine.
   2. Distinct cytokine receptor signaling pathways can converge at the same cellular response (eg, NFκB activation).
I. Cytokines can **amplify** a biological response by inducing additional cytokine synthesis (Figure 12–1).
J. Certain cytokines **antagonize** the effects of other cytokines.
   1. IFN-γ inhibits the effects of IL-4 on B cells.
   2. IL-10 and transforming growth factor (TGF)-β antagonize the effects of IFN-γ on macrophages.
K. There are dedicated **inhibitors** of cytokines.
   1. **IL-1 receptor antagonist (IL-1ra)** is produced by the same cells that secrete IL-1 and binds to the same receptor.
   2. The amino-terminus of TGF-β maintains the secreted cytokine in a latent form until it is removed by proteolysis.

TUBERCULOSIS IN RHEUMATOID ARTHRITIS

- **Rheumatoid arthritis (RA)** is an autoimmune disease characterized by inflammation of the joints and a progressive loss of joint function.
- New therapies for RA include the use of anticytokine reagents to block the action of TNF-α or IL-1β.
- For example, Etanercept is a recombinant protein consisting of a portion of a TNF receptor (p75) fused to the Fc portion of human immunoglobulin (Ig) G to prolong its circulating half-life.

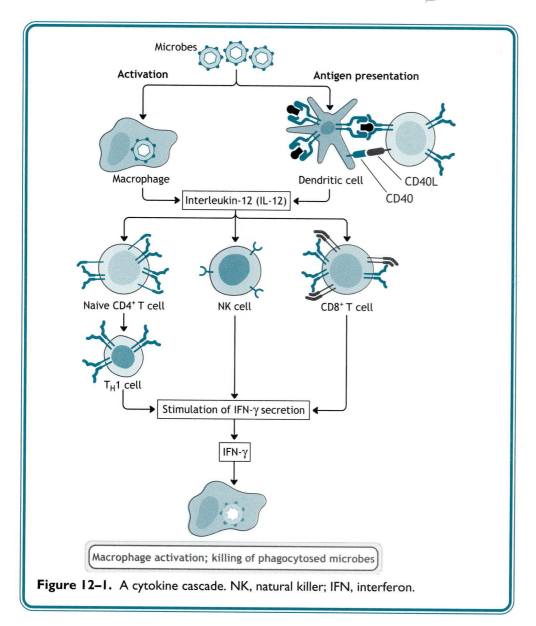

Figure 12–1. A cytokine cascade. NK, natural killer; IFN, interferon.

- *Combining an anti-TNF-α and an anti-IL-1β drug in these patients increases the risk of pulmonary tuberculosis.*
- *This finding emphasizes the importance of using anticytokines under conditions that inhibit inflammation without impairing innate host defenses.*

II. Macrophages, natural killer (NK) cells, and NKT cells are important sources of proinflammatory cytokines that also mediate innate immunity (Table 12–2).

Table 12–2. Cytokines that mediate innate immunity and acute inflammation.[a]

Biological Function	Important Cytokines	Specific Examples
Leukocyte adhesion	TNF-α	Induces ICAM-1 expression on endothelium
Chemotaxis	TGF-β IL-8	Recruits blood monocytes Recruits blood neutrophils
Induction of other inflammatory mediators	IFN-γ	Promotes macrophage activation for IL-1 and TNF-α production
Fever induction	IL-1β	Activates cells of the hypothalamus
Acute phase protein synthesis	IL-6, IL-1, TNF-α	Activates hepatocytes and Kupffer cells to produce fibrinogen and complement components
Oxidant production	TNF-α IFN-γ	Activates neutrophils for superoxide production Activates macrophages for NO production
Inhibition of immunity	IL-10, TGF-β	Inhibits TNF-α synthesis by IFN-γ-activated macrophages
Apoptosis	TNF-α LT, IL-2	Apoptosis of tumor cells Activation induced cell death in T cells

[a]TNF, tumor necrosis factor; ICAM, intercellular adhesion molecule; TGF, transforming growth factor; IL, interleukin; IFN, interferon; LT, leukotriene.

A. These cells bear receptors that recognize both conserved microbial structures and endogenous ligands derived from damaged host cells.
1. Macrophages express Toll-like receptors (TLRs) (Table 1–2).
2. NK cells and NKT cells recognize exogenous and endogenous ligands from infected, stressed, or injured host cells (Table 10–4).

B. The cytokines produced by these cells signal **danger** to phagocytes and endothelial cells.
1. **TNF-α** has the following functions.
   a. It stimulates the expression of **adhesion molecules** and **integrins** on endothelial cells and leukocytes, respectively.
   b. It primes **neutrophils** and **macrophages** for respiratory bursts and NO production.
   c. It induces the synthesis of **acute phase proteins**.
   d. It induces **apoptosis** through its death domain-containing receptor.

2. **IL-1β** has the following functions.
   a. It is redundant with TNF-α (Table 12–1).
   b. It synergizes the effects of TNF-α.
   c. It induces **fever** by stimulating the hypothalmus.
3. **IL-12** has the following functions.
   a. It coactivates NK cells and T cells.
   b. It coinduces **IFN-γ production** and cytotoxicity by NK cells and NKT cells.
   c. It induces the differentiation of CD4⁺ Th1 cells.
4. **IFN-γ** (type II interferon) has the following functions.
   a. It **activates macrophages**.
   b. It induces the production of other **proinflammatory cytokines**, including TNF-α, IL-1β, IL-6, and the chemokine CCL4.
   c. It promotes **major histocompatibility complex (MHC) class II** gene expression.
   d. It promotes the differentiation of CD4⁺ Th1 cells.
5. **Type I interferons (IFN-α/β)** have the following functions.
   a. They **block virus replication** by autocrine signaling.
   b. They increase **MHC class I expression**.
   c. At low levels they **coactivate macrophages**.
   d. At high concentrations they inhibit macrophage and lymphocyte activation.
6. **Chemokines** have the following characteristics.
   a. Chemokines are chemotactic cytokines that are produced rapidly in response to the danger signals associated with infection and inflammation.
   b. They **attract cells** to sites of infection or inflammation.

C. The proinflammatory effects of these cytokines are balanced by **antiinflammatory cytokines (eg, IL-10), cytokine-binding proteins**, and **receptor antagonists** (see above).

D. The amount of a cytokine that is secreted determines its overall effects.
   1. In **low to moderate levels** of production, proinflammatory cytokines initiate important innate mechanisms of host defense.
   2. When produced at **high concentrations**, proinflammatory cytokines cause the **systemic inflammatory response syndrome (SIRS)**.
      a. **Sepsis** is a form of SIRS initiated by infection (Chapter 11).
      b. SIRS can be induced by any stimulus that activates large numbers of inflammatory cells and mediators.

SYSTEMIC INFLAMMATORY RESPONSE SYNDROME (SIRS)

- SIRS is defined as a constellation of clinical signs and symptoms, including **hyperthermia** (> 38°C) or **hypothermia** (< 36°C), **tachycardia** (> 90 bpm), **tachypnea** (> 20 breaths/min), and/or **altered white blood cell (WBC) counts** (> 12,000/μL or < 4,000/μL).
- **Septicemia** (microbes in the blood stream) and microbial **toxemia** (toxins in the blood stream) are among the leading causes, in which case the syndrome is called **sepsis** or **septic shock**.
- Regardless of the initiating event, proinflammatory cytokines play a central role.
- Multiorgan dysfunction, including acute respiratory distress syndrome, is a common sequela.
- Mortality rates when multiorgan failure is present approach 90%.

E. Cytokines of innate immunity are secreted in a temporal sequence.
   1. TNF-α is produced early and promotes leukocyte localization at sites of infection.
   2. Chemokines are produced early as a means of recruiting leukocytes to affected tissue sites.
   3. Cytokines that activate phagocytes (eg, IFN-γ) are produced somewhat later.

III. Cytokines of adaptive immunity provide coactivating signals for lymphocytes and regulate antigen-presenting cells.

A. Cytokines that induce **humoral immunity** are concerned with B cell recruitment, activation, growth, and differentiation.
   1. IL-2 from CD4$^+$ Th1 cells induces B cell proliferation and increases Ig and J chain synthesis.
   2. IL-4 from **CD4$^+$ Th2 cells** promotes **Ig class switching** to IgE, induces the differentiation of naive CD4$^+$ T cells into **Th2 cells**, and **antagonizes** IFN-γ-driven Ig class switching to IgG$_3$.
   3. IL-5 and **TGF-β** promote the synthesis of IgA by B cells.
   4. The chemokine **CCL7** directs antigen-stimulated B cells to T-dependent areas of the lymph nodes.
   5. The coactivating effects of IL-4 on B cells are balanced by the inhibitory effects of IFN-γ.

B. Cytokines that promote **cellular immunity** induce the activation, growth, and/or differentiation of T cells, NK cells, NKT cells, and macrophages.
   1. IL-2 has the following characteristics.
      a. It is an autocrine **growth factor** for many CD4$^+$ and CD8$^+$ T cells.
      b. It enhances the cytotoxic activity of NK cells and conventional CD8$^+$ T cells.
      c. It costimulates T cells for the production of IL-4, IL-5, and IFN-γ.
      d. It promotes the development of **Treg cells**.
      e. It induces autocrine **activation-induced cell death** in T cells (Chapter 11).
   2. IFN-γ has the following characteristics.
      a. It is primarily produced by CD4$^+$ Th1 cells and CD8$^+$ T cells during adaptive immune responses.
      b. It activates macrophage **intracellular killing** of microbes.
      c. It increases both class I and class II **antigen presentation** pathways by increasing MHC, transporter associated with antigen processing (TAP) protein, the proteasome subunits, and HLA-DM expression (Chapter 7).
      d. It promotes Th1 polarization by naive CD4$^+$ T cells.
      e. It inhibits Th2-associated humoral immunity.

DEFICIENCY IN IFN-γ SIGNALING

CLINICAL CORRELATION

- *Genetic deficiencies have been described for either chain of the heterodimeric IFN-γ receptor.*
- *Patients with these defects are susceptible to infections by viruses and* Mycobacterium *and* Salmonella *species, two intracellular bacterial pathogens.*
- *The same phenotype is associated with defects in the expression of either IL-12 or the IL-12 receptor, illustrating the importance of IL-12 as an inducer of IFN-γ.*

   3. Lymphotoxin (LT or **TNF-β)** has the following characteristics.
      a. It is produced by activated T cells.

b. It has many of the same proinflammatory and apoptosis-inducing effects as TNF-α.

    4. TGF-β is chemotactic for blood monocytes.

IV. Cytokines, referred to as **colony-stimulating factors (CSFs)** or **poietins**, coordinate the diverse process of **hematopoiesis** (Figure 12–2).

    A. Stem cell factor (SCF) and **IL-3** have broad growth-promoting effects on multiple blood cell lineages.

    B. Lymphopoiesis is regulated by **IL-7** (T and B cells), **IL-2** (T cells), and **IL-15** (NK cells).

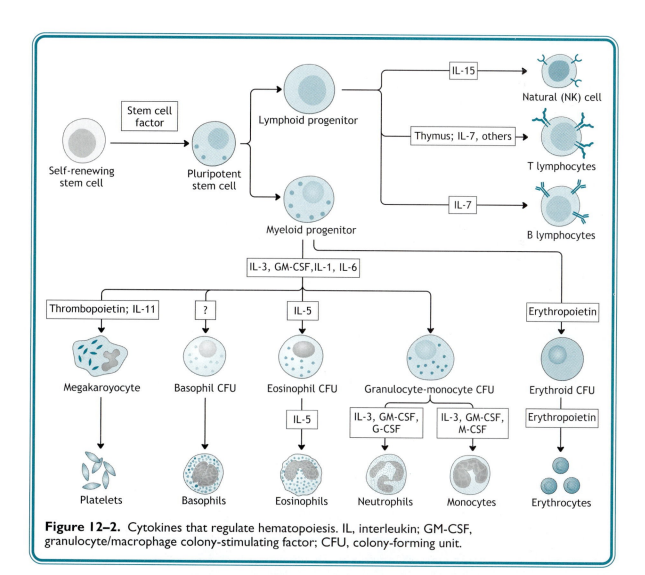

Figure 12–2. Cytokines that regulate hematopoiesis. IL, interleukin; GM-CSF, granulocyte/macrophage colony-stimulating factor; CFU, colony-forming unit.

C. Myelopoiesis is controlled by **erythropoietin (EPO)**(erythrocytes), **thrombopoietin** (platelets), **IL-5** (eosinophils), **granulocyte/macrophage (GM)-CSF** and **G-CSF** (neutrophils), and GM-CSF and **M-CSF** (monocytes).

D. Recombinant CSFs are now used routinely to correct certain defects in hematopoiesis.

ANEMIA AND ERYTHROPOIETIN

- **Anemia** is a reduction in red cell mass and has a number of causes, including depressed erythropoiesis.
- Chronic diseases, such as renal failure, malignancy, autoimmune diseases, and certain infections, are often accompanied by decreased EPO production.
- For the treatment of anemia associated with end-stage renal disease, EPO has replaced blood transfusions as a therapy.
- Repeated transfusions of whole blood to prospective renal transplant recipients often immunizes them against the HLA antigens of the blood donors.
- This can result in antibody-mediated hyperacute rejection of a subsequent transplant (Chapter 17).

V. Chemokines, a diverse family of chemotactic cytokines, regulate normal cell traffic, tissue architecture, and inflammatory cell recruitment.

A. Chemokines establish a chemical concentration gradient that is sensed by the cell.

B. They induce the expression of leukocyte integrins that mediate leukocyte binding to and migration between vascular endothelial cells.

C. Chemokines induce cytoskeletal changes that mediate cell migration.

D. The two largest chemokine families are designated **CCL#** or **CXCL#** (distinguished by the arrangement of their cysteine residues)(Table 12–3).

    1. CCL chemokines attract monocytes, lymphocytes, and eosinophils.

    2. Most CXCL chemokines attract neutrophils, although some act on lymphocytes.

Table 12–3. Examples of CC and CXC chemokines and their receptors.[a]

Chemokine (Ligand)	Also Known as	Receptors	Cells Attracted
CCL4	MIP-1β	CCR5	T cells, NK cells, DC, and monocytes
CCL11	Eotaxin	CCR3	Eosinophils, basophils, Th2 cells
CXCL2	ENA-78	CXCR2	Neutrophils
CXCL8	IL-8	CXCR1, CXCR2	Neutrophils
CXCL10	IP-10	CXCR3	T cells

[a]MIP, macrophage inflammatory protein; NK, natural killer; DC, dendritic cells; ENA-78, epithelial neutrophil-activating protein 78; IL, interleukin; IP-10, interferon-γ-inducible protein 10.

E. Chemokine production is induced by a variety of immune and inflammatory stimuli, including TNF-α, IL-1β, IFN-γ, and IL-4.

F. Cellular responses to chemokines are mediated by seven-transmembrane, G protein-coupled cell surface receptors designated CCR# or CXCR#.

G. Some chemokine receptors serve as coreceptors for virus entry.
1. HIV-1 uses both CCR5 and CXCR4 as coreceptors with CD4.
2. The tissue distribution of these chemokine receptors specifies the tissue tropism of a particular HIV-1 clone.

VI. Cytokines activate cells by binding to high-affinity receptors (Table 12–4)

A. Cytokine receptors induce gene expression by activating latent cytosolic transcription factors.

B. The **type I (hematopoietic) receptors** activate the **Janus kinase (Jak)** signaling pathway.
1. Jak is a family of receptor-associated tyrosine kinases that is activated upon receptor clustering.
2. Jak phosphorylation of cytokine receptors recruits **signal transducers and activators of transcription (STAT)** peptides.
3. Jak phosphorylates STAT peptides and the peptides dimerize.
4. Dimerization of STAT results in nuclear localization, DNA binding, and transcriptional activation.

Table 12–4. Cytokine receptor families.[a]

Receptor Family	Ligands	Signaling Mechanism
Type I (hematopoietic)	IL-2, 3, 4, 5, 6, 7, 12, 13, 15, G-CSF, GM-CSF	Jak activation of latent, preformed STAT transcription factors
Type II (interferon-like)	IFN-α/β, IFN-γ, IL-10	Jak activation of latent, preformed STAT transcription factors
TNF	TNF, LT, CD40L, FasL	Binding of adapter proteins and activation of NFκB and AP-1 Binding of adapter proteins and activation of caspases
Ig superfamily	IL-1, M-CSF, SCF	Binding of adapter proteins and activation of latent NFκB
Seven-transmembrane G protein coupled	Chemokines	GTP exchange Activation of PLC and PI3K

[a]IL, interleukin; Jak, Janus kinase; STAT, signal transducers and activators of transcription; GM-CSF, granulocyte/macrophage colony-stimulating factor; IFN, interferon; TNF, tumor necrosis factor; LT, leukotriene; SCF, stem cell factor; PLC, phospholipase C; PI3K, phosphatidylinositol-3'-kinase.

5. The receptors for **IL-2, 3, 4, 6, 7, 12, and 13, G-CSF, and GM-CSF** utilize the Jak/STAT pathway for signaling.

C. Type II interferon-like receptors for IFN-α/β, IFN-γ, and IL-10 also signal through Jak/STAT.

D. The **TNF receptor** family utilizes adapter proteins to activate diverse signaling pathways.

    1. When adapter proteins with **death domains** are recruited, caspase activation signals apoptosis.

    2. When adapters without death domains are recruited, **kinase activation** results in the activation of NFκB.

E. The **Ig superfamily** of receptors, such as the IL-1 receptor, activates NFκB using specialized adapter proteins (eg, MyD88) (Figure 1–3).

F. G protein-coupled **chemokine receptors** signal through phospholipase C (PLC), phosphatidylinositol-3´-kinase (PI3K), and guanosine triphosphate (GTP) ex change proteins.

G. Different forms of the IL-2 receptor show different affinities for IL-2.

    1. Resting T cells, B cells, and NK cells express the β and γc chains of IL-2R, which shows a moderate affinity for IL-2 (10^{-9} M).

    2. Activated T cells express an additional α chain in their IL-2R, which increases receptor affinity to 10^{-11} M.

COMMON γ CHAIN (γC) DEFICIENCY

- *Whereas cytokine deficiencies are extremely rare, an X-linked recessive cytokine receptor defect is the most common cause of **severe combined immune deficiency**.*
- *Mutations in the common γ chain (γc) impair the development of T cells and NK cells, because the receptors for IL-2, IL-4, IL-7, and IL-15 share the γc subunit.*
- *The resulting T⁻B⁺NK⁻ phenotype places these infants at risk for infections with intracellular pathogens.*

CLINICAL PROBLEMS

A 5-month-old male patient presents with enlarged lymph nodes, and a biopsy shows acid-fast bacteria, a feature of infections with mycobacteria. The patient shows a normal complete blood count (CBC) and differential, normal T and B cell subsets by flow cytometry, and normal serum Ig levels when referenced to age-matched controls.

1. For which of the following cytokines would a mutation in its receptor explain this clinical picture?

    A. IL-1

    B. IL-2R

    C. TNF-α

    D. IFN-γ

    E. IL-10

2. Which of the following additional cytokine deficiencies would produce a similar phenotype?

 A. IL-12 deficiency

 B. IL-7 deficiency

 C. IL-15 deficiency

 D. SCF deficiency

 E. IL-4 deficiency

A patient who received a cardiac transplant from an unrelated donor is given the drug cyclosporine to control rejection of his allograft.

3. Which of the following receptors signals through an intermediate that is sensitive to the drug cyclosporine?

 A. IL-1 receptor

 B. IL-2 receptor

 C. T cell receptor (TCR)

 D. TLR4

 E. CXCR4

The blood lymphocytes of a 6-month-old child with recurrent, complicated viral and fungal infections do not respond normally to IL-2 and IL-4 in vitro. The patient currently has thrush and a cytomegalovirus (CMV) infection. The patient has a single gene mutation that explains all of these findings.

4. Which of the following immune functions might you expect to be **normal** in this child?

 A. Neutrophil ingestion of bacteria

 B. NK cell killing of virus-infected cells

 C. T cell activation by antigen + antigen-presenting cells (APCs)

 D. Ig class switching by B cells cultured with the patient's T cells

 E. Killing of CMV-infected cells by CD8$^+$ cells

A menstruating teenager presents to the emergency room in shock and is diagnosed as suffering from toxic shock syndrome secondary to a vaginal infection with the bacterium *Staphylococcus aureus*.

5. Which of the following cytokines is both key to host defense against this organism and a central mediator of toxic shock pathogenesis?

 A. IL-10

 B. TNF-α

 C. IL-3

 D. TGF-β

 E. IL-5

ANSWERS

1. The correct answer is D. Mutations in the IFN-γR result in susceptibility to intracellular pathogens (bacterial and fungal) early in life. This probably results from the failure to activate infected macrophages, a cell type commonly infected by these pathogens.

2. The correct answer is A. Because of its role as a coinducer of IFN-γ, IL-12 is also essential for the induction of cellular immunity to intracellular bacterial pathogens, such as the mycobacteria. Defects in the IL-12R produce a similar clinical picture.

3. The correct answer is C. None of the cytokine receptors signals through a cyclosporine-sensitive pathway, although the production of IL-2 and IL-4 by activated T cells is inhibited by the drug. Cyclosporine inhibits calcineurin and the activation of nuclear factor of activated T cells (NFAT), which induces transcription of genes in T and B cells.

4. The correct answer is A. The only known gene defect that could interfere with responses to both IL-2 and IL-4 is a mutation in the γc chain of the IL-2R and IL-4R. This defect also blocks IL-15R signaling, which would result in an absence of NK cells. The overall phenotype in the periphery would be T⁻B⁺NK⁻.

5. The correct answer is B. TNF-α is a key mediator of both toxic (Chapter 6) and septic shock (Chapters 1 and 12). Toxic shock is initiated when superantigens produced by certain microbes, including the gram-positive *Staphylococcus*, activate Th cells and macrophages by cross-linking TCRs to MHC class II molecules. Massive cytokine production results when both cell types are activated.

CHAPTER 13
IMMUNE TISSUE INJURY

I. **Robust immune responses, even to relatively nonthreatening antigens, can cause host tissue damage.**

A. An **allergy** (or **hypersensitivity**) is an adaptive immune response to an environmental antigen that damages tissues and causes organ dysfunction.
1. Allergy is mediated by specific antibodies and/or effector T cells.
2. The signs and symptoms of allergy include watery eyes, runny nose, sneezing, coughing, wheezing, and pruritic (itchy) hives.
3. An **allergen** is an antigen that can produce these signs and symptoms (Table 13–1).
4. Typical allergens include pollens, animal dander, insect venoms, and foods.

B. **Atopic allergies** are familial, rapid, and strong reactions mediated by immunoglobulin (Ig) E.
1. **Atopy** is a heritable predisposition to produce IgE antibodies and other allergic mediators in response to environmental antigens.
2. Atopic conditions are more common in developed countries with high levels of air pollutants and closed living spaces.
3. Common manifestations of atopic allergies are **allergic rhinitis, allergic asthma, atopic dermatitis,** and **allergic anaphylaxis.**

C. **Anaphylaxis** is a systemic form of allergy involving the cardiovascular, respiratory, cutaneous, and gastrointestinal systems.
1. **Anaphylactic shock** includes hypotension, tissue hypoxia, and the loss of consciousness.
2. **Anaphylactoid shock** is similar in its presentation, but is not mediated by IgE.
   a. IgG antibodies mediate systemic anaphylactoid reactions.
   b. Complement-mediated mast cell activation produces anaphylaxis-like symptoms.

D. Allergies can develop to inhaled, ingested, or injected antigens or antigens encountered by contact with the skin (Table 13–1).
1. Tree and grass pollens induce seasonal **rhinitis** and **conjunctivitis.**
2. Peanuts, shellfish, eggs, and dairy products often cause **food allergies.**
3. Insect and snake venoms and injected drugs (eg, penicillin) can cause **allergic anaphylaxis.**
4. Plant resins (eg, poison ivy pentadecacatechol), industrial chemicals, and metals can cause **allergic contact dermatitis.**

Table 13–1. Common allergies and allergens.

Clinical Manifestations	Typical Sources of Allergens
Atopic allergic rhinitis and allergic asthma	Tree and grass pollens, mold spores, mites in house dust, pet dander
Allergic gastroenteritis	Food products (milk, eggs, shellfish)
Occupational allergies	Pharmaceuticals, organic and inorganic compounds, enzymes, microbial agents, dyes, plant products, shellfish, animal products
Urticaria and anaphylaxis	Foods (shellfish, nuts, seeds), drugs (polypeptide hormones, enzymes, haptenic drugs, opiates), insect venoms
Contact dermatitis	Nickel and other metals, formaldehyde, epoxy resins, neomycin cream, benzocaine, plant resins
Drug allergies	β-Lactam antibiotics, NSAIDs[a]

[a]NSAIDs, nonsteroidal antiinflammatory drugs.

   E. Gell and Coombs first described the four major mechanisms of immune tissue injury that underlie human hypersensitivies (Table 13–2).
      1. The mechanisms differ in terms of the nature of the antigen, the immune components involved in their pathogenesis, and the nature and onset of clinical symptoms.
      2. Antigenic specificity is mediated by antibodies and/or T cells.
      3. Tissue damage results from the activation of complement, mast cells, neutrophils, macrophages, or lymphocytes.
      4. Immune tissue injury mediated by the **innate immune system** is not included in the Gell and Coombs classification scheme.
   F. Immune tissue injury mediated by adaptive immunity requires two phases.
      1. Sensitization occurs on first exposure to the allergen (Figure 13–1).
         a. Antibody production and/or the proliferation of T cells occur during the sensitization phase.
         b. Antibody can either bind to cellular Fc receptors or remain in the circulation, depending on Ig class.
         c. Tissue damage is not generally seen during the sensitization phase.
      2. During the **elicitation phase**, antibodies or immune T cells recognize the allergen and trigger effector mechanisms.
         a. For example, large numbers of memory CD4[+] Th1 cells are activated to produce cytokines.
         b. Allergen–antibody complexes activate complement to produce inflammatory peptides.

Table 13–2. The Gell and Coombs classification of immune tissue injury mediated by adaptive immunity.[a]

Type	Time from Exposure to Response	Form of the Antigen	Antibodies	Cellular Immune Mediators	Soluble Immune Mediators	Clinical Examples
I	Minutes	Protein or hapten-protein	IgE	Mast cells, basophils, eosinophils	Histamine, proteases, eicosinoids, cytokines, chemokines	Atopic allergies Allergic asthma
II	Hours to days	Cell or tissue bound	IgG or IgM	Neutrophils	C3b, C3a, C4a, C5a	Transfusion reactions
III	Hours to days	Soluble	IgG or IgM	Neutrophils	C3b, C3a, C4a, C5a	Lupus nephritis
IV	Days	MHC-bound peptide	None	APCs, T cells, NK cells, macrophages	IL-2, IFN-γ, chemokines	Allergic contact dermatitis

[a]Ig, immunoglobulin; MHC, major histocompatibility complex; APC, antigen-presenting cells; NK, natural killer; IL, interleukin; IFN, interferon.

    c. Mast cells with IgE antibodies bound to their surface Fc receptors degranulate when allergen is encountered.

G. Innate immunity also causes localized tissue damage, but does not require a prior exposure to the foreign agent (ie, a sensitization phase).
    1. The tissue damage seen in **septic arthritis** is caused by the activation of neutrophils recruited to an infected joint.
    2. Innate immune tissue injury can be elicited by relatively nontoxic microbial products, such as bacterial DNA or cell wall lipopolysaccharide (LPS).
        a. **Sepsis** is an acute systemic inflammatory response to infection mediated by **danger signals** and the excessive production of inflammatory mediators.
        b. Responses to components of nonpathogenic microbial flora can induce organ-specific inflammatory tissue damage.
            (1) **Crohn's disease** is thought to be initiated by innate immune responses to intestinal microbial flora.
            (2) **Ulcerative colitis** appears to involve a similar imbalance of the mucosal immune system.

CROHN'S DISEASE

- *Crohn's disease (CD) is a chronic transmural inflammation of the large and small bowel that begins with the loss of epithelial barrier function in the intestine.*
- *Some CD patients have mutations in the Nod2 antimicrobial protein, which diminishes their ability to clear bacteria that breach the epithelium.*

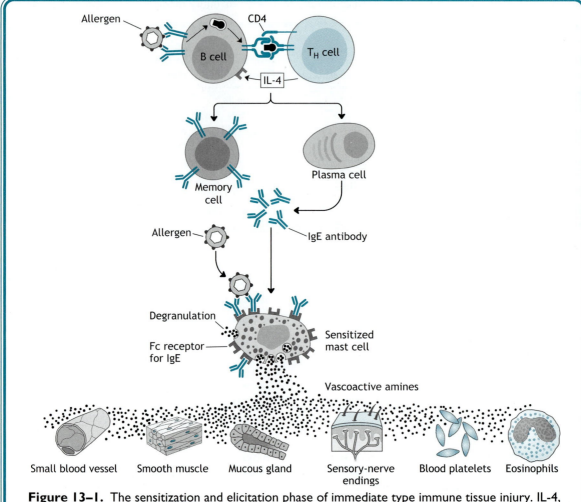

Figure 13–1. The sensitization and elicitation phase of immediate type immune tissue injury. IL-4, interleukin 4; IgE, immunoglobulin E.

- *Aberrant innate immune responses develop in the gastrointestinal tract to the intestinal flora.*
- *Activated macrophages and Th1 cells produce excessive interleukin (IL)-12, interferon (IFN)-γ, and tumor necrosis factor (TNF)-α.*
- *Sustained macrophage and neutrophil activation contributes to chronic inflammation.*
- *Blocking the action of TNF-α with monoclonal antibodies to the cytokine has proven effective in the treatment of CD.*

II. Type I (immediate-type) immune tissue injury (Table 13–2) is a rapid response to environmental antigens mediated by IgE antibodies and vasoactive inflammatory mediators released by mast cells.

A. The antigens that elicit these responses are **proteins** or **haptens** (eg, drugs) that can bind to proteins.
   1. The allergens are presented by major histocompatibility complex (MHC) class II molecules and activate **CD4⁺ Th2 cells**.
   2. Th2 cells produce IL-4 and IL-13, which induce class switching to IgE.

B. The propensity to make high-titer IgE antibodies to environmental allergens is, in part, genetically determined.
   1. Multiple genes control susceptibility to allergy and asthma.
   2. Among the traits that appear to be genetically controlled are total IgE levels, Th2 polarization, and mast cell and eosinophil growth.

C. Allergen-specific IgE antibodies bind to **Fcε receptor I (FcεRI)** on tissue **mast cells**.
   1. FcεRI is a very high-affinity receptor (K_d = 10 pM).
   2. The activation of mast cells through FcεRI requires receptor cross-linking by multideterminant antigens.
   3. Because the antibodies displayed on mast cells are specific for many different epitopes, polyvalent protein antigens can cross-link surface FcεRI molecules.

D. The tissue distribution and density of mast cells as well as the surface density of FcεRI determine the distribution of tissue injury.
   1. The route of immunization (eg, respiratory versus gastrointestinal) determines the local distribution of antibody specificities on tissue mast cells.
   2. Mucosal and connective tissue mast cells produce distinct patterns of inflammatory mediators.

HYPER-IgE SYNDROME

- **_Hyper-IgE syndrome_** or **_Job's syndrome_** *is an immune deficiency characterized by recurrent and severe staphylococcal skin abscesses and pneumonia.*
- *Th1:Th2 imbalance results in a decreased production of IFN-γ, a cytokine that normally inhibits Th2 responses, such as switching to IgE production.*
- *These patients can also show pruritic dermatitis, but increased allergy is not common, despite exceedingly high serum IgE levels (> 2000 IU/mL).*

E. Signaling through FcεRI results in three mechanisms of inflammatory mediator release (Figure 13–2).
   1. Preformed mediators stored in cytoplasmic granules are released when mast cells **degranulate**.
      a. Allergen binding triggers FcεRI clustering.
      b. Phospholipase Cγ (PLCγ) is recruited to the immunotyrosine activation motifs (ITAMs) of the FcεRI and is activated.
      c. Protein kinase C (PKC) is then activated by diacylglycerol and phosphorylates myosin light chains.
      d. Cytoskeleton changes are induced that promote granule exocytosis and the release of granule constituents.
         (1) The preformed vasoactive amine **histamine** (Table 13–3) is released.
         (2) Heparin, the proteases **chymase** and **tryptase**, and **chemotactic peptides** that recruit neutrophils and eosinophils are also released from granules.
      e. Degranulation can be inhibited by maintaining elevated levels of **intracellular cyclic AMP (cAMP)**.

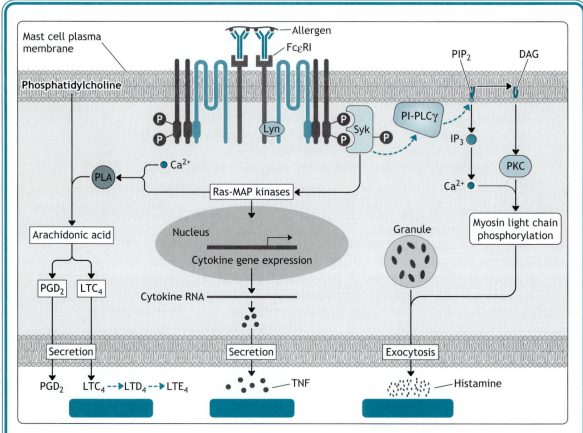

Figure 13–2. Fcε receptor I (FcεRI) signaling in mast cells. PIP$_2$, phosphatidylinositol 4,5-biphosphate; DAG, diacylglyceride; PLCγ, phospholipase Cγ; IP$_3$, inositol 1,4,5-triphosphate; PLA$_2$, phospholipase A$_2$; MAP, mitogen-activated protein; PKC, protein kinase C; PGD$_2$, prostaglandin D$_2$; LT, leukotriene; TNF, tumor necrosis factor.

2. FcεRI cross-linking also activates **phospholipase A$_2$** (PLA$_2$).
  a. PLA$_2$ cleaves phosphatidylcholine to form **arachidonic acid**.
  b. Arachidonic acid is metabolized by the **cyclooxygenase** and **lipoxygenase** pathways to form **prostaglandins (PGs)** and **leukotrienes (LTs)**, respectively.
3. The de novo expression of **cytokine genes** is induced by the activation of transcription factors.
  a. **Nuclear factor of activated T cells (NFAT), nuclear factor-κB (NFκB),** and **AP-1** are activated in mast cells.
  b. The genes for **IL-3, IL-4, IL-5, IL-6, IL-13,** and **TNF-α** are transcribed.

Table 13–3. Inflammatory mediators derived from activated mast cells.[a]

Preformed or Newly Synthesized	Mediators	Proinflammatory Effects	Mast Cell Signaling Intermediates
Preformed mediators	Histamine Heparin Tryptase Chymase E-CFA N-CFA	Itchy sensation, vasodilation, increased vascular permeability, bronchoconstriction, mucus secretion, leukocyte chemotaxis, gut peristalsis	PLCγ, Ca^{2+} mobilization, PKC activation, myosin phosphorylation, granule exocytosis
Newly synthesized mediators	PAF, prostaglandins (PGD$_2$), leukotrienes (LTC$_4$) IL-3, IL-4, IL-5, IL-6, TNF-α, eotaxin	Vasodilation, increased vascular permeability, bronchoconstriction, eosinophil chemotaxis, mucus secretion, platelet aggregation, ICAM-1 expression, mast cell growth, Th2 cell differentiation	PLA$_2$ activation, arachidonic acid, COX-2 NFκB, NFAT, and AP-1 activation

[a]E-CFA, eosinophil chemotactic factor of anaphylaxis; N-CFA, neutrophil chemotactic factor of anaphylaxis; PLCγ, phospholipase Cγ; PKC, protein kinase C; PAF, platelet-activating factor; IL, interleukin; TNF, tumor necrosis factor; ICAM, intercellular adhesion molecule; PLA$_2$, phospholipase A$_2$; COX, cyclooxygenase; NFκB, nuclear factor κB; NFAT, nuclear factor of activated T cells.

IgE-INDEPENDENT MAST CELL ACTIVATION

- *Several agents can activate mast cells without binding as allergens to cell surface IgE.*
- *Certain **drugs** (morphine, codeine, calcium ionophores, vancomycin, radiocontrast agents) can activate mast cells directly and induce anaphylaxis.*
- *The **anaphylatoxins** C3a, C4a, and C5a trigger mast cell degranulation.*
- *The **neuropeptides** substance P and somatostatin mediate cholinergic triggering of asthma by activating mast cells.*
- *Lectins, such as those found in some foods, can bind carbohydrate residues on IgE and induce adverse reactions to foods.*

    F. The signs and symptoms of allergy reflect the action of mast cell mediators on target tissues (Table 13–3).

       1. Most of the inflammatory effects of **histamine** in allergy are mediated through binding of histamine to H$_1$ **histamine receptors**.

         a. H$_1$ receptors are G protein coupled and activate adenylate cyclase.

         b. Adenylate cyclase activation leads to a *transient* increase in intracellular cAMP concentrations.

       2. The effects of histamine depend on the cell type affected.

a. Histamine relaxes smooth muscle cells in peripheral blood vessels causing **vasodilation**.

    b. Histamine induces **bronchospasms** in the lungs and **peristalsis** in the intestines by stimulating smooth muscle contraction.

    c. Histamine causes contraction of vascular endothelial cells resulting in **increased vascular permeability** and edema.

3. Tryptase and **chymase** are serine proteases stored in granules.

    a. The circulating levels of tryptase are a clinical measure of recent mast cell degranulation.

    b. Tryptase induces **mucus secretion** in the lungs.

    c. Tryptase can activate certain matrix metalloproteases.

    d. Tryptase cleaves plasminogen to form plasmin, which cleaves C3.

4. Mast cell granules contain two chemotactic peptides.

    a. Eosinophil chemotactic factor of anaphylaxis (E-CFA) attracts eosinophils to the lung in asthma and to the intestine in certain parasitic infections.

    b. Neutrophil chemotactic factor of anaphylaxis (N-CFA) recruits neutrophils that contribute to tissue damage.

5. Proteoglycans, including **heparin** and **chondroitin sulfate**, are granule constituents to which other mast cell mediators are bound.

SYSTEMIC ALLERGIC ANAPHYLAXIS

CLINICAL CORRELATION

- *The allergens that typically induce systemic anaphylaxis include drugs, insect venoms, and certain foods.*
- *Key target organs include the cardiovascular, pulmonary, gastrointestinal, and cutaneous systems.*
- *Typical signs and symptoms of anaphylactic shock include generalized pruritis, apprehension, hypotension, abdominal cramping, tachycardia, tachypnea, and hives.*
- *Timely injection of epinephrine is life saving.*
- *Drugs that inhibit the late phase of anaphylaxis are essential to avoid a secondary shock response several hours later.*

6. Three groups of **lipid mediators** contribute to allergic responses.

    a. Platelet activating factor (PAF) is derived from the PLA_2-mediated hydrolysis of membrane phospholipids.

       (1) PAF is produced by mast cells, basophils, and endothelial cells.

       (2) PAF induces **vasodilation, bronchoconstriction,** and increased **vascular permeability**.

    b. PGs are derived from the metabolism of arachidonic acid via the **cyclooxygenase (COX) pathway**.

       (1) **COX-2** is the principal mast cell cyclooxygenase.

       (2) PGD_2 is the principal prostaglandin produced.

       (3) PGD_2 causes **vasodilation** and **bronchoconstriction**.

    c. LTs are derived from arachidonic acid by the **lipoxygenase pathway**.

       (1) LTC_4, LTD_4, and LTE_4 are the principal leukotriene mediators of allergy.

       (2) LTC_4 is produced by mucosal mast cells, but not connective tissue mast cells (eg, in the skin).

       (3) LTC_4 is a major cause of **bronchoconstriction**.

7. **Cytokines** are expressed by mast cells following transcription.
   a. **IL-3** and **IL-4** promote the growth of mast cells.
   b. **IL-4** and **IL-13** induce B cell class switching to IgE.
   c. **IL-5** is a chemotactic factor for eosinophils.
   d. **IL-4** promotes eosinophil growth.
   e. **TNF-α** facilitates leukocyte chemotaxis by inducing vascular intercellular adhesion molecule (ICAM)-1 and leukocyte integrin expression.
   f. Cytokines mediate many of the **late-phase** allergic responses.

ALLERGIC ASTHMA

- *The allergic form of asthma is caused by IgE-mediated immunity to inhaled allergens.*
- *Th2 polarization probably begins early in life.*
- *Asthmatic "attacks" can be triggered by either intrinsic signals (eg, cold outside air or exercise) or extrinsic signals (ie, allergens).*
- *Chronic mast cell activation leads to persistent mediator release, bronchoconstriction (chest tightness), mucus secretion, and eosinophil recruitment and activation.*
- *Eosinophils damage the mucosal epithelium, cause perivascular edema, and initiate lung tissue remodeling.*
- *Mucus plugging of the bronchi results in the hyperinflation of the lungs, an inability to expire air, and expiratory wheezing.*
- *Early intervention is designed to diagnose and treat the underlying allergic conditions.*
- *As the disease progresses, more aggressive treatment to control chronic inflammation (eg, corticosteroids) must be considered.*

   G. The proper diagnosis of atopic allergies requires a careful patient history and allergy skin testing.
      1. The diagnostic gold standard for allergy is the **skin test**.
         a. Allergen injected into the skin induces histamine release, localized edema (**wheal**), and a zone of erythema (**flare**) within 20 minutes.
         b. Negative and positive controls (eg, saline and histamine, respectively) are essential to validate the test.
      2. The **radioallergosorbant test (RAST)** is useful for measuring the circulating levels of IgE antibodies to known allergens (Chapter 5).

HAY FEVER

- *Allergic rhinitis or hay fever can be a perennial or seasonal condition.*
- *For example, in the Midwest, ragweed pollenosis shows a well-delineated season with symptoms appearing first in mid-August and lasting through the first frost.*
- *Rhinitis presents as sneezing, nasal congestion, and watery, itchy eyes.*
- *Typical allergens include pollens, fungal spores, animal dander, and house mites.*
- *The accurate identification of the allergen requires a careful patient history combined with skin testing using standardized allergens.*

   H. Prophylaxis and treatment of allergic conditions take many forms.
      1. The first approach to prophylaxis is to avoid the allergen.
      2. **Immunotherapy** is an effort to divert the immune system away from IgE-mediated triggering of mast cells.

a. The patient receives repeated intradermal injections of the allergen over several months.

b. Some patients produce IgG and IgA antibodies that compete with allergenic IgE.

c. The IgE antibody levels in some patients decrease by unknown mechanisms.

d. A Th2 to Th1 shift in immunity to the allergen may occur.

3. Antibodies to the Fc portion of IgE (omalizumab) are beneficial for treating severe allergic asthma (Table 13–4).

a. The antibodies decrease circulating levels of IgE.

b. They decrease the density of FcεRI on tissue mast cells.

4. **Desensitization** is a therapy designed to establish a temporary block of allergen-induced mast cell mediator release.

a. Desensitization is most often used when no alternative therapy exists for a patient with a drug allergy.

b. The patient is given the allergenic drug in incrementally increasing doses beginning with a subclinical dose.

c. Desensitization probably results from the gradual, controlled release of mast cell mediators.

d. The desensitized state persists only while the drug is given.

Table 13–4. Pharmacological treatment of allergy.[a]

Group	Examples	Mechanisms of Action	Clinical Uses
Anti-IgE	Omalizumab	Decreasing circulating IgE	Asthma
Antihistamines	Diphenhydramine, fexofenadine	H_1 receptor antagonists	Allergic rhinitis, urticaria, anaphylaxis
β_2-Agonists	Epinephrine, albuterol	β_2-Adrenergic agonist	Anaphylaxis, asthma, urticaria
NSAIDs	Indomethacin	Blocks PG synthesis	Urticaria
Corticosteroids	Beclomethasone, methylprednisolone	Blocks PLA_2 and cytokine expression	Allergic rhinitis, asthma, anaphylaxis
Mast cell stabilizers	Cromolyn sodium	Prevents granule fusion	Allergic rhinitis Asthma
Methylxanthines	Theophylline	Inhibits phosphodiesterase	Asthma
Leukotriene receptor antagonists	Zafirlukast	Blocks LT action	Asthma

[a]IgE, immunoglobulin E; NSAIDs, nonsteroidal antiinflammatory drugs; PG, prostaglandin; PLA_2, phospholipase A_2; LT, leukotriene.

5. Inhibiting mast cell degranulation is effective against allergy.
   a. Cromolyn sodium inhibits Ca^{2+} influx, an important step in FcεRI signaling.
   b. Theophylline maintains high intracellular cAMP levels in mast cells.
   c. Nonsteroidal antiinflammatory drugs (NSAIDs) (eg, indomethasone) inhibit arachidonic acid metabolism.
   d. Hydrocortisone acts at multiple steps in mast cells.
      (1) It inhibits histamine synthesis from histidine.
      (2) It inhibits the activation of PLA_2.
      (3) The drug blocks NFκB activation by increasing the expression of its inhibitor IκB.

FOOD ALLERGIES

- *Food intolerance can be IgE dependent or IgE independent.*
- *Most adults show the IgE-dependent form, whereas significant numbers of infants or children have food intolerance that is not IgE mediated.*
- *Common allergens include proteins of peanuts, soybeans, shellfish, milk, and eggs.*
- *Oropharyngeal symptoms (pruritis and urticaria in the mouth) appear first followed by nausea, cramping, vomiting, flatulence, and diarrhea.*
- *Urticarial rashes and even anaphylaxis can result from allergic reactions to foods.*
- *IgA deficiency increases the childhood risk of developing IgE-mediated food allergies.*

6. Some drugs block the effects of allergic mediators.
   a. The β-adrenergic receptor agonist **epinephrine** blocks histamine action.
   b. Epinephrine is life saving in acute allergic anaphylaxis.
   c. The $β_2$-receptor agonist **albuterol** is an effective bronchodilator used for the treatment of allergic asthma.
   d. Antihistamines include the H_1 receptor antagonists (eg, **diphenhydramine** and **chlorpheniramine**).
   e. Leukotriene receptor antagonists are used to treat asthma.
   f. Hydrocortisone and other corticosteroids also block inflammatory gene expression in target cells.

III. Type II (cytotoxic) immune tissue injury results from the recognition of cell- or tissue-bound antigens by IgG and IgM antibodies (Table 13–2).

A. Tissue damage generally requires hours or days to become evident.

B. IgM and **IgG antibodies** activate **complement** through the classical pathway.
   1. Tissue damage can result from the formation of the **membrane attack complex** C5b-9.
   2. C5a is **chemotactic** for neutrophils.
   3. C3a, C4a, and C5a are **anaphylatoxins** that directly activate mast cells.
   4. Phagocytic cells can cause tissue damage when they attach to IgG- or iC3b-coated tissues and cells.

C. Anemia is a common effect of cytotoxic immune tissue injury directed toward erythrocyte antigens.
   1. Transfusion reactions result when mismatched blood is transfused to a patient with a preformed antibody.

2. Rh disease of the newborn is due to maternal IgG antibodies that cross the placenta and bind to fetal Rh antigens.

3. A number of **autoimmune diseases** (eg, Coombs-positive hemolytic anemias and thrombocytopenias) are mediated by host antibodies reacting with autoantigens (Chapter 16).

D. Damage to solid tissues and extracellular matrix is also mediated by cytotoxic immune tissue injury.

    1. Hyperacute graft rejection is mediated by anti-HLA antibodies.

    2. Autoantibodies in **Goodpasture syndrome** react with type IV collagen of the glomerular basement membrane.

E. The **diagnosis** of type II immune tissue injury is often based on detecting an abnormal distribution of IgG.

    1. The Coombs test detects Ig on erythrocytes.

    2. Immunofluorescence can detect IgG deposition within tissues.

IV. Type III (immune complex) tissue injury results when soluble antigen–antibody complexes form in the blood and deposit in tissues.

A. Immune complex deposition in the kidneys causes **nephritis**.

B. Immune complexes in the joints result in **arthralgia** and **arthritis**.

C. Immune complexes in the skin cause a range of lesions, including **rashes**.

D. Immune complex deposition in blood vessel walls causes **vasculitis, purpura,** and **edema**.

E. IgG-containing immune complexes activate complement in tissues.

    1. C5a attracts neutrophils to sites of immune complex deposition.

    2. iC3b serves as an adhesion ligand promoting neutrophil binding.

    3. The membrane attack complex damages cells.

    4. Immune complex formation often causes a transient decrease in the serum levels C1, C2, C3, and C4.

F. Diagnosis involves the detection of antibodies in the serum or affected tissues.

SERUM SICKNESS

- *Serum sickness* *was first described in the preantibiotic era as a reaction to horse antitoxins given repeatedly for the treatment of toxin-mediated infectious diseases.*

- *The condition can arise after antibody production to either protein [eg, intravenous immunoglobulins (IVIG), foreign monoclonal antibodies, vaccines] or nonprotein (eg, penicillin or sulfonamides) antigens.*

- *Serum sickness typically becomes evident 1–3 days after exposure to the antigen.*

- *Signs and symptoms include fever, rash, hypotension, anaphylactoid purpura, lymphadenopathy, myalgia, arthralgia, and nephritis.*

- *The treatment of **anaphylactoid syndrome** is the same as that for anaphylaxis, ie, discontinuance of the antigen and administration of epinephrine, antihistamines, and corticosteroids.*

V. Type IV (delayed-type) immune tissue injury is a manifestation of cell-mediated immunity to haptens or protein antigens.

A. The immunologically specific component of **delayed-type hypersensitivity (DTH)** is the Th1 cell, rather than antibody.

1. Allergens must be proteins or chemically reactive groups capable of binding co-valently to proteins.
2. Important cytokines include **IL-1, TNF-α, IL-2, IL-12, IFN-γ**, and the **CCL** group of chemokines (Chapter 12).

B. Host tissue damage is mediated by cytotoxic T lymphocytes, natural killer (NK) cells, macrophages, and a range of soluble inflammatory mediators.
1. Macrophages and Th1 cells produce the proinflammatory cytokines IL-1, IL-2, IFN-γ, and TNF-α.
2. Macrophages produce eicosinoids (LTs and PGs), hydrolytic enzymes, and re-active oxygen species.

C. The important clinical manifestations of type IV hypersensitivity show delayed onset (2–3 days) and include **contact dermatitis**.
1. Plant resins (eg, poison ivy pentadecacatechol), metals (eg, nickel) and chemi-cals (eg, cosmetics) cause a variety of rashes.
2. Industrial exposure to certain drugs, including antibiotics, can cause type IV hypersensitivities.

D. Delayed-type hypersensitivity (DTH) skin lesions are initially characterized by their **indurated** (firm) nature, rather than the edematous (fluid-filled) lesions of atopic allergy.

E. The diagnosis of allergic contact dermatitis is aided by the **patch test**.
1. Solutions of test allergens are placed on absorbent skin patches.
2. The extent of induration and erythema beneath each patch is determined 48–72 hours later.

CLINICAL PROBLEMS

A 44-year-old school teacher who paints houses in the summer presents in early June with erythematous, indurated, and blistering lesions limited to his hands and forearms. The le-sions typically appear each summer within several days of beginning to use painting prod-ucts, including solvents and epoxy resins. He indicates that he does not wear protective gloves when working with these chemicals. The lesions disappear several weeks after he re-turns to his teaching position in the fall.

1. Which of the following represents a likely step in the pathogenesis of this disease?

   A. Activation of C1

   B. Chemotaxis of neutrophils

   C. Induction of IgE antibodies

   D. Antigen presentation by the MHC class II pathway

   E. Immune complex deposition

2. Which of the following test results would best fit the clinical findings in this case?

   A. A positive skin test after 20 minutes with a dilute solution of epoxy resin

   B. A positive skin patch test with a dilute solution of epoxy resin

C. Decreased serum levels of C1, C2, C3, and C4

D. A decreased CD4:CD8 ratio

E. Elevated serum tryptase

Jim received penicillin for pneumonia several years ago and presented last week with what appeared to be an allergic reaction to the drug when it was taken for a sinus infection. The next day after beginning oral penicillin, Jim's eyelids became puffy and his abdomen was covered with itchy, nearly confluent hives. After the administration of diphenhydramine and hydrocortisone his condition improved. Laboratory tests performed on his acute serum showed an elevated level of tryptase and decreased C1 and C3. A skin test with penicillin was negative.

3. Which of the elements of this case suggests this reaction was caused by circulating IgG antibody–drug complexes, rather than IgE antibody to penicillin?

A. His plasma tryptase level was elevated.

B. His symptoms were corrected by administering antihistamines.

C. His C1 and C3 levels were decreased.

D. His skin lesions were pruritic (itchy).

E. He showed evidence of altered vascular permeability.

Jesse is a 10-year-old child who complains of chest tightness and wheezing after gym class and upon exposure to cold outside air. He experiences sneezing, nasal itching, and nasal congestion indoors and following contact with his friend's dog. His allergist has determined by skin testing that he is allergic to oak pollen, Bermuda grass, house dust, and dog dander. His pulmonary function tests indicate a forced expiratory volume in 1 second (FEV_1) < 60% of the expected value for his age and a peak flow rate of 180 L/min (normal > 350 L/min).

4. Which of the following drugs would be most beneficial in alleviating Jesse's pulmonary symptoms?

A. Albuterol

B. Anti-TNF-α monoclonal antibody

C. IVIG

D. Cyclosporin

E. Recombinant IL-4

Anna is a 7-year-old child who presents with itchy, erythematous, indurated lesions on her forearms and legs 3 days after a camping trip with her classmates. Her mother treats Anna with antihistamines, which reduces the itching sensation, but does not correct the skin lesions.

5. What additional therapy would probably benefit this child?

A. Albuterol by inhaler

B. Topical corticosteroids

C. Epinephrine

D. Anti-IgE

E. Cromolyn sodium

ANSWERS

1. The correct answer is D. The patient's history suggests this is an occupational exposure to a contact allergen in solvents. The indurated nature of the lesions suggests mononuclear cell infiltration into the skin, and the time necessary for their development (several days) is consistent with allergic contact dermatitis.

2. The correct answer is B. The standard diagnostic test for allergic contact dermatitis is the patch test. Dilute solutions of well-standardized test allergens are available that can be placed on the skin. It is essential that the test samples be dilute enough to not cause primary irritant reactions on the skin.

3. The correct answer is C. This clinical picture would normally be attributed to a type I hypersensitivity reaction mediated by IgE antibodies. However, two aspects of his reaction suggest this is not the pathogenic mechanism. First, he did not test positive to the allergen in an immediate-type skin test. Second, his complement levels were decreased, suggesting the activation and depletion of complement by circulating antigen–antibody complexes. It should also be noted that his symptoms did not appear immediately.

4. The correct answer is A. Albuterol is a β_2-receptor agonist and is used as a bronchodilator in asthma. It acts by antagonizing histamine-induced signaling in the lung. Jesse's pulmonary dysfunction results from his lungs being hyperinflated. In addition, his breathing is impaired by bronchoconstriction and mucus plugging.

5. The correct answer is B. The time to onset of symptoms and the indurated nature of the lesions suggest this is a case of poison ivy rash. Corticosteroids are administered topically to inhibit macrophage and lymphocyte activation in the skin, which are two features of delayed-type contact dermatitis.

CHAPTER 14
PROTECTIVE IMMUNITY AND VACCINES

I. **Only a subset of the immune responses we make to microbes is protective.**

  A. **Neutralizing antibodies** are very effective at controlling infectious agents and limiting the effects of their toxins.

   1. Antibodies can prevent viral entry into and uncoating within host cells.

   2. Neutralizing antibodies against microbial exotoxins (eg, tetanus toxin) block toxin binding to host cells.

   3. **Seroconversion** refers to the appearance of antibodies to a microbial pathogen in a patient.

     a. Seroconversion can aid in the diagnosis of a specific infectious disease.

     b. Alternatively, seropositivity may simply indicate a prior encounter with the organism (or a cross-reacting species), rather than an ongoing or recent infection.

  B. The **clearance** of extracellular microbes is primarily mediated by opsonophagocytosis.

   1. Opsonins include antibodies, complement peptides, and soluble pattern recognition molecules (Chapter 1).

   2. Opsonic receptors also initiate microbial killing mechanisms.

  C. **Killing** of microbes can occur either outside or inside immune cells.

   1. Extracellular pathogens that are small enough to be phagocytized (eg, bacteria) are killed within phagocytic cells.

   2. Large extracelluar pathogens (eg, filamentous fungi) are killed when phagocytes adhere to the surface of the microbe.

  D. The **resolution** of an infection requires the complete eradication of the infectious agent.

   1. Patients with underlying cellular immune defects often do not resolve infections well.

   2. Infections often reappear in these patients after antimicrobial therapy is discontinued.

   3. Unresolved infections can also persist in normal individuals if the microbe (eg, *Mycobacterium tuberculosis*) establishes a **latent infection**.

  E. Innate and adaptive immunity provide distinct forms of protection.

   1. **Innate immunity** to microbes is essential early in an infection and lowers the early microbial burden in the host.

2. Innate immunity is more important in immunologically naive hosts (eg, neonates) who lack **adaptive immunity** to the pathogen.
3. Adaptive immunity arises late in primary infections and often mediates resolution of infections.
4. Adaptive immunity can mediate lifelong specific protection against a particular pathogen.
5. Adaptive immunity is the objective of our current **vaccines**.

WORLDWIDE INFECTION RATES

- *Each year infectious diseases account for one-third of all deaths worldwide.*
- *Infectious diseases that are prevalent in developing countries are often not common in the United States.*
- *For example, tens of millions of individuals worldwide have schistosomiasis, leishmaniasis, and tuberculosis.*
- *Malaria, tuberculosis, and AIDS each causes several million deaths each year.*
- *Because of the complexity of these organisms and the relatively low level of research on these pathogens, effective vaccines have been slow to emerge.*

II. The specific protective immune response to a microbial pathogen depends on the life-style of the microorganism (Tables 14–1 and 14–2).

    A. Protection against **extracellular pathogens** (eg, most bacteria) requires killing of the microbe within an intracellular organelle by phagocytic cells.

    B. Large **extracellular pathogens** (eg, filamentous fungi) are killed when phagocytes direct these antimicrobial responses to the extracellular environment.

    C. Protective responses to **obligate intracellular microbes** limit microbial replication or kill the infected cell as a means of destroying the microbe.

    D. While in the extracellular phase of their life cycle, **obligate and facultative intracellular microbes** can be neutralized and cleared from the host by antibodies and complement.

III. At least eight distinct immune mechanisms are known to provide protection against microbial pathogens.

    A. Membrane lysis is most effective against microbes with outer membranes (eg, gram-negative bacteria) or lipid envelopes (eg, enveloped viruses).
        1. Among the gram-negative bacteria, *Neisseria* species are among the most susceptible to complement-mediated membrane attack.
        2. Antimicrobial peptides appear to act by damaging the outer membranes of bacteria.

    B. Opsonophagocytosis is primarily directed at extracellular bacteria, fungi, and parasites.
        1. Most opsonic receptors signal phagocytes for increased antimicrobial activity.
        2. Pyogenic bacteria are particularly susceptible to opsonophagocytic clearance and killing.

    C. Microbial killing by neutrophils is essential for elimination of extracellular microbes.

Table 14–1. Protective immune responses to infectious agents.[a]

Protective Mechanisms	Immune Components	Groups of Pathogens	Specific Pathogens
Membrane attack	Defensins, cathelicidins Complement	Gram-negative bacteria	*Pseudomonas aeruginosa Neisseria* species
Opsonophagocytosis	Neutrophils, macrophages Opsonic receptors (CR3, FcR) and ligands (iC3b, IgG)	Extracellular pyogenic bacteria and yeasts	*Staphylococcus, Streptococcus, Pseudomonas* species
Intracellular killing	Phagolysosomes; reactive oxygen	Extracellular bacteria and yeasts	Many catalase-negative bacteria and fungi
Toxin neutralization	IgM, IgG, IgA antibodies Immune complex clearance	Exotoxin-producing microbes	*Clostridium tetani, Staphylococcus aureus, Escherichia coli*
Virus neutralization	IgM, IgG, IgA antibodies Phagocytic cells, mucus	Respiratory and gastrointestinal viruses	Rhinoviruses, adenoviruses, rotaviruses
Extracellular killing	Neutrophils, macrophages	Filamentous fungi, parasites	*Histoplasma capsulatum, Candida albicans*
Macrophage-mediated intracellular killing	Th1 cells, NK cells, IFN-γ, nitric oxide	Obligate or facultative intracellular pathogens	*Mycobacterium tuberculosis, Listeria monocytogenes, Candida albicans, Histoplasma capsulatum*
Cytotoxic T cell killing	CD8+ T cells, MHC class I, CD4+ Th cells, and IL-2	Viruses and many intracellular bacteria and fungi	Herpes simplex virus, *Listeria monocytogenes*
Eosinophil-mediated cytotoxicity	Eosinophils, IgE antibodies, FcεR	Intestinal parasites (helminths)	*Taenia saginata*
Inhibition of intracellular replication	Type I interferons	Most viruses	Herpesviruses
NK cell-mediated cytotoxicity	NK cells, MHC class I	Many viruses	Herpesviruses

[a]Ig, immunoglobulin; NK, natural killer; IFN, interferon; MHC, major histocompatibility complex.

Table 14–2. Important protective immune components organized by microbe class.[a]

Immune Component	Extracellular Bacteria	Intracellular Bacteria	Viruses	Fungi	Parasites
Antibody	++	Minimal	++	–	++
Complement	++	Minimal	+ (enveloped)	–	–
Neutrophils	++	– or +	–	+	– (eosinophils)
Th2 cells	++	–	++	–	–
Th1 cells	–	++	++	++	++
Macrophages	+	++	+	++	++
Cytotoxic T cells	–	+	++	–	
NK cells	++ (cytokines)	+ (cytokines)	+ (lysis)	Unknown	Unknown

[a]NK, natural killer.

1. **Reactive oxygen species** (eg, hydrogen peroxide) mediate killing of many aerobic microbes.
2. A more limited range of microbes (eg, *Lysteria, Mycobacterium* species) is killed by **reactive nitrogen species** (eg, nitric oxide).
3. For the killing of anaerobic microbes, oxidants are less important than antimicrobial peptides and lysosomal hydrolases.

D. Intracellular microbes (eg, *Mycobacterium, Legionella, Listeria, Salmonella,* and *Francisella* species) that replicate within mononuclear phagocytes are particularly susceptible to **Th1-type cellular immunity**.
   1. Macrophage activation by Th1 cytokines is a key step.
   2. A combination of reactive oxygen and nitrogen metabolites and oxygen-independent mediators mediates killing.

E. **Toxin neutralization** is important in decreasing the severity of infectious diseases mediated by endo- and exotoxins.

F. **Virus neutralization** is particularly important in blocking virus attachment to mucosal surfaces and in clearing viruses from the blood stream.
   1. Secretory immunoglobulin (Ig) A antibodies protect against inhaled and ingested viruses.
   2. IgG antibodies reduce viremia and block virus spread.
   3. Antibodies are particularly important for viruses (eg, rabies, polio) that require hematogenous dissemination.

G. Cytotoxic T cells (CTL) provide protection against intracellular pathogens whose antigens are presented by major histocompatibility complex (MHC) class I molecules.

1. Most virus-infected cells are susceptible to CTL attack.

2. Microbes that block the class I pathway of antigen presentation (eg, herpesviruses) can evade CTL-mediated clearance.

3. Intracellular bacteria that escape the phagosome (eg, *Listeria, Francisella*) are also subject to detection by CTL.

H. Natural killer (NK) cells also protect against pathogen-infected host cells.

1. NK cells can recognize and kill infected host cells in which the microbe has inhibited **MHC class I** expression.

2. NK cells produce **type I interferons** (IFN-α, β) early in infection.

   a. IFN-α, β establishes an antiviral state within infected cells.

   b. IFN-α, β induces RNase L and protein kinase R, which degrade viral mRNA and block translation, respectively.

I. Eosinophils use **IgE antibodies** to attack extracellular parasites (eg, intestinal worms) by antibody-dependent cellular cytotoxicity (ADCC).

III. The nature of opportunistic infections in immunocompromised patients can reveal important protective immune responses (Table 14–3).

A. Infections with intracellular pathogens are common in patients lacking **Th1 cell, CTL, NK cell,** or **macrophage** functions.

B. Microbes that replicate within the cytosol (eg, viruses) are particularly problematic for patients with **CTL** or **MHC class I** defects.

Table 14–3. Common infections in the immunocompromised patient.[a]

	T Cells	B Cells	Phagocytic Cells	Complement
Bacteria	Mycobacterium, Listeria	Stahpylococcus, Streptococcus, Haemophilus	Staphylococcus, Streptococcus, Haemophilus	Staphylococcus, Streptococcus, Neisseria
Fungi	Candida, Histoplasma, Pneumocystis		Aspergillus, Candida	
Viruses	CMV, HSV, VZV, EBV, JC	Enteroviruses, influenza, RSV		
Principal mechanisms	Macrophage, NK cell, and CTL activation	Virus neutralization, opsonophagocytosis	Phagocytosis, intracellular killing	Membrane attack, chemotaxis and opsonophagocytosis

[a]CMV, cytomegalovirus; HSV, herpes simplex virus; VZV, varicella-zoster virus; EBV, Epstein–Barr virus; RSV, respiratory syncytial virus; NK, natural killer; CTL, cytotoxic T cell.

C. Opportunistic infections with extracellular bacteria (eg, *Staphylococcus aureus*) and some cytolytic viruses (eg, influenza viruses) are common in **antibody-deficiency** states.

D. Extracellular bacteria and fungi commonly infect patients with **neutrophil** defects, including deficiencies in oxidant production or granule expression.

E. Patients with **complement** deficiencies cannot lyse gram-negative bacteria and enveloped viruses or clear extracellular microbes.

IV. Microbial immune evasion mechanisms have evolved to circumvent the most important protective responses by the host.

   A. Antigenic variation allows bacteria, viruses, and parasites to avoid immune recognition.

   1. Point mutations in antigenic proteins **(antigenic drift)** occur in influenza and human immunodeficiency virus (HIV)-1 by error-prone nucleic acid replication.

   2. Other organisms, including *Neisseria gonorrhea* and *Trypanosoma cruzii*, scramble the genes that encode their major surface antigens.

   3. More substantial changes in antigens **(antigenic shift)** occur by genetic recombination between related viruses.

   B. Adopting an **intracellular life cycle** is a microbial response to immune elimination mediated by antibody and complement.

   1. The host response to this microbial strategy has been to evolve CTL and NK cells capable of recognizing a microbe-infected cell.

   2. Antigen presentation can be viewed as a host adaptation to intracellular microbial parasitism.

   C. Disguising microbial antigens prevents immune recognition and attack.

   1. Schistosomes coat themselves with host MHC molecules.

   2. *Plasmodium* species (etiological agents of malaria) infect erythrocytes that do not express MHC molecules.

   3. Many bacteria (eg, *Streptococcus pneumoniae* and *Haemophilus influenzae*) express thick polysaccharide capsules that disguise their more antigenic cell wall components.

   4. The long polysaccharide chains of bacterial lipopolysaccharide (LPS) molecules direct complement activation away from the bacterial outer membrane.

ANTIGENIC SHIFT IN THE INFLUENZA A VIRUS

- *The influenza A virus is responsible for periodic worldwide pandemics.*
- *Protective immunity to this virus depends on the production of neutralizing antibodies to two surface glycoproteins, neuraminidase (N) and hemagglutinin (H).*
- ***Antigenic drift** is the gradual change in the N and H serotypes by mutation.*
- *Regular monitoring of the N and H gene sequences determines the serotype of the predominant influenza virus each flu season, and an appropriate vaccine is produced.*
- *Occasionally, a major **antigenic shift** occurs due to reassortment of genomes between different influenza virus strains, including those of animals.*
- *The 1957 "Asian flu" pandemic resulted from the sudden emergence of new H and N serotypes by genetic reassortment between antigenically distinct influenza viruses.*

D. **Suppression of the immune response** is another common approach to evasion.
  1. HIV-1 infects and depletes $CD4^+$ T cells.
  2. Herpesviruses, HIV-1, and adenoviruses inhibit MHC expression or transporter associated with antigen processing (TAP) function and thereby depress CTL activation.
  3. Many viruses produce proteins that mimic inhibitory cytokines or bind to activating cytokines (eg, Epstein–Barr virus and poxviruses, respectively).
  4. Protein A produced by staphylococci binds IgG Fc regions.
  5. *Streptococcus pyogenes* produces a C5a peptidase.
  6. *N gonorrhea* produces a protease that degrades secretory IgA.
  7. *Legionella* and *Listeria* species avoid intracellular killing by blocking phagosome–lysosome fusion or escaping from the phagosome, respectively.

V. Effective vaccines augment protective host responses to infection.

A. Vaccines do not typically prevent infections, although they reduce the severity of infectious diseases.

B. Most existing vaccines are **preemptive**; they must be given prior to infection (Table 14–4).

Table 14–4. Recommended immunizations for children.[a]

Vaccine	Birth	1 mo	2 mo	4 mo	6 mo	12 mo	15 mo	18 mo	24 mo	4–6 yr
Hepatitis B										
Diphtheria, tetanus, pertussis										
Haemophilus influenzae type b										
Inactivated poliovirus										
Measles, mumps, rubella										
Varicella										
Pneumococcal conjugate										
Influenza					Annual					
Hepatitis A									At risk	At risk

[a]Adapted from www.cdc.gov/nip/recs/child-schedule.htm#printable. The different shades denote the different number of immunizations (eg, children should receive three immunizations with the hepatitis B vaccine).

1. Only a few vaccines (eg, rabies, hepatitis) are **therapeutic vaccines** that can be used to treat an infected patient.

2. Rabies is a slowly progressing infection that does not outpace the immune response.

C. All existing vaccines are directed at **epitopes**, not microbial patterns, and induce adaptive immunity.

D. We have very few vaccines against complex microbes (eg, parasites).

E. Most of our best vaccines induce neutralizing antibodies.

F. Routine **pediatric vaccines** (Table 14–4) are designed to prevent life-threatening infectious diseases of childhood.

1. These diseases typically outpace the ability of the neonate to mount an adequate protective immune response.

2. Immunization is also valuable when the dose of a microbial toxin (eg, tetanus toxin) sufficient to cause disease is far less than the immunizing dose.

3. Some vaccines (eg, *H influenzae* type b conjugate vaccine) are designed to elicit opsonic IgG antibodies that would not normally be made during an infection in children.

G. **Practical issues dictate the design and use of vaccines.**

1. Live attenuated vaccines can cause disease in an immunodeficient individual and should be avoided.

2. Repeated immunizations are required to attain high-titered, long-lasting protective immunity or to compensate for antigenic shift.

3. Multiple immunizations are necessary to induce Ig isotype switching (eg, IgG antibody formation).

COMMON COLDS IN CHILDREN

CLINICAL
CORRELATION

- *Children normally contract five or six colds (upper respiratory tract infections) each year.*
- *This frequency is increased by exposure to day care centers and cigarette smoke, allergies and asthma, cystic fibrosis, congenital immune defects, and ciliary dyskinesia.*
- *Several hundred different viruses can cause the common cold, including the rhinoviruses, influenza viruses, adenoviruses, and respiratory syncytial virus.*
- *The development of a vaccine for this disease has been hampered by the wide variety of antigenically distinct agents responsible for these infections.*

4. The design of a vaccine should theoretically reflect the principal protective response desired in the host (Table 14–5).

a. Immunization against intracellular pathogens requires a live vaccine that duplicates the intracellular infection.

b. **Live attenuated vaccines** are useful when inducing a CTL response.

c. **Polyvalent vaccines** (eg, *Neisseria* species) are useful when multiple serotypes of a pathogen cause disease.

d. **Subunit vaccines** (eg, hepatitis B) are effective when inducing immunity to surface antigens or toxins.

e. **Conjugate vaccines** (eg, *H influenzae* type b) promote the production of IgG antibodies to T-independent epitopes.

f. **Mucosal immunization** (eg, influenza nasal vaccine) can protect against respiratory or gastrointestinal pathogens.

Table 14–5. Types of vaccines.

Type of Vaccine	Examples
Live attenuated	Oral polio, varicella; mumps, measles, rubella, bacillus Calmette–Gúerin (BCG)
Killed or inactivated	Inactivated polio
Subunit	Diphtheria toxoid, tetanus toxoid
Recombinant subunit	Hepatitis B
Conjugate	*Haemophilus influenzae* type b, *Streptococcus pneumoniae*
Polyvalent	*S pneumoniae*

NOVEL VACCINE STRATEGIES

- *Molecular biological techniques provide the means for isolating genes from microbial pathogens and expressing them in relatively safe viral vectors.*
- *This permits the construction of **polyvalent vaccines** carrying genes for a large number of microbial antigens.*
- ***Adjuvant** activity can be included by also expressing genes for human cytokines (eg, switch cytokines or Th1 cell-inducing cytokines) and costimulatory molecules.*
- ***DNA vaccines** are another approach that could be used to induce T cell-mediated immunity by directing microbial protein expression associated with host MHC.*

CLINICAL PROBLEMS

A 15-month-old child is seen by his pediatrician for a cough, congestion, and fever of 39°C. He has a rapid pulse, appears ill, and is unresponsive. His white blood cell count is elevated. His mother seems unsure of his immunization history, but recalls only two visits to the county health clinic for immunizations. The pediatrician prescribes the antibiotic ampicillin, and the child's condition improves substantially over the next few days.

1. A routine pediatric vaccine for which of the following pathogens might have prevented this condition?

   A. Rabies

   B. Poliovirus

   C. *Legionella pneumophila*

   D. *Haemophilus influenzae* type b

   E. Hepatitis B

Harry is aware that he has a congenital deficiency of the C6 complement peptide.

2. For which of the following infectious agents is Harry particularly susceptible?

   A. *Streptococcus pneumoniae*

   B. *Neisseria meningitidis*

   C. *Clostridium tetani*

   D. *Mycobacterium tuberculosis*

   E. *Clostridium difficile*

Donald has a defect in his IFN-γ receptor resulting from an inherited mutation in one of the receptor-encoding genes.

3. Which of the following pathogens would most likely cause recurrent infections in this child?

   A. *Pseudomonas aeruginosa*

   B. *Streptococcus pyogenes*

   C. *Staphylococcus aureus*

   D. *Legionella pneumophila*

   E. *Neisseria meningitidis*

A 1-day-old child born of an uncomplicated full-term pregnancy presents with jaundice. The mother is Rh⁺, and the newborn is not anemic. Suspecting a congenital virus infection, viral serology on a sample of the child's serum is ordered. High-titered IgG antibodies to cytomegalovirus are found.

4. What can be concluded from these clinical and laboratory findings?

   A. The patient has a congenital cytomegalovirus (CMV) infection.

   B. The infant suffers from Rh disease of the newborn.

   C. The child should be immunized immediately to limit CMV infection.

   D. The infant should be given broad-spectrum antibiotics.

   E. The positive CMV serology reflects the immune status of the mother.

Milind is a 56-year-old immigrant from India who is brought to the emergency room with a cough that produces blood-containing sputum. He has a positive skin test with tuberculin purified protein derivative (PPD), and his chest x-ray shows lesions typical of mycobacterial pneumonia. He indicates that he was immunized with bacillus Calmette–Gúerin (BCG) as a child.

5. What is the nature of this vaccine?

   A. Subunit vaccine

   B. Conjugate vaccine

   C. Live attenuated vaccine

   D. Recombinant vaccine

   E. Polyvalent vaccine

ANSWERS

1. The correct answer is D. *H influenzae* is a gram-negative bacterium that can cause mild nasopharyngeal infections. In young children, these conditions can progress to meningitis, and vaccination has proven effective at reducing morbidity and mortality. Multiple immunizations in children are recommended by 15 months of age (Table 14–4).

2. The correct answer is B. *Neisseria* species are among the most susceptible to complement-mediated lysis by the C5b-9 membrane attack complex due to the structure of their outer membranes. The other organisms listed do not have classic outer membranes.

3. The correct answer is D. Only *Legionella pneumophila* is an intracellular pathogen. Defective IFN-γ signaling would impair Th1 cellular immunity, especially the activation of macrophages. This bacterium establishes an intracellular infection within resting macrophages and is killed when macrophages become activated.

4. The correct answer is E. High-titered antibodies to CMV in a newborn's serum most likely reflect IgG that has crossed the placenta from the mother. Vaccinating the child at this point would not limit the infection, and there currently is no CMV vaccine.

5. The correct answer is C. The BCG strain is a live bovine mycobacterium that induces cross-protective immunity to other *Mycobacterium* species in humans. Its effectiveness derives from its ability to establish life-long Th1-type cellular immunity against mycobacterial antigens, but protection is variable among vaccines.

CHAPTER 15
IMMUNE DEFICIENCY STATES

I. Primary immune deficiency diseases in human beings are generally rare, inherited conditions affecting a defined immune component (Figure 15–1 and Table 15–1).

    A. The term **congenital** is also used to describe these diseases, because they are inherited and become apparent early in life.

    B. Recurrent infections are the most common clinical presentation.

        1. The nature of the infections in an immunocompromised patient can provide important clues for establishing a diagnosis.

            a. These infections are often with **opportunistic pathogens**, which do not pose problems for healthy individuals.

                (1) Opportunistic agents generally show low virulence.

                (2) Many opportunistic microbes are normal flora.

            b. The infections may resist aggressive antimicrobial therapy or may not **resolve** (Chapter 14) after the completion of the therapy.

            c. The infection may **progress more rapidly** than it would in an immunocompetent individual of the same age.

            d. The course of the infections may be unusual in **severity** or **organ involvement**.

            e. The infections may occur much **earlier in life** (eg, during the first week) than would be seen in a normal child.

            f. The infections may show **delayed onset** in infancy (eg, after 6 months of life), reflecting the normal decline of maternal antibody acquired during pregnancy.

            g. Similar infections may have occurred **within a family**, especially among male infants.

            h. The infections may follow shortly **after immunization** with a live vaccine.

        2. In adults, recurrent infections more often indicate an **acquired** or **secondary immune deficiency**.

            a. A history of **high risk behavior for human immunodeficiency virus (HIV)-1 infection** (intravenous drug abuse, unprotected sex with an infected partner) supports a diagnosis of an acquired immune deficiency.

            b. Chemotherapy for cancer or **occupational exposure** to ionizing radiation increases the risk of immunodeficiency.

            c. Patients who are receiving **immunosuppressive therapy** for autoimmune disease or following transplantation are at risk for recurrent infections.

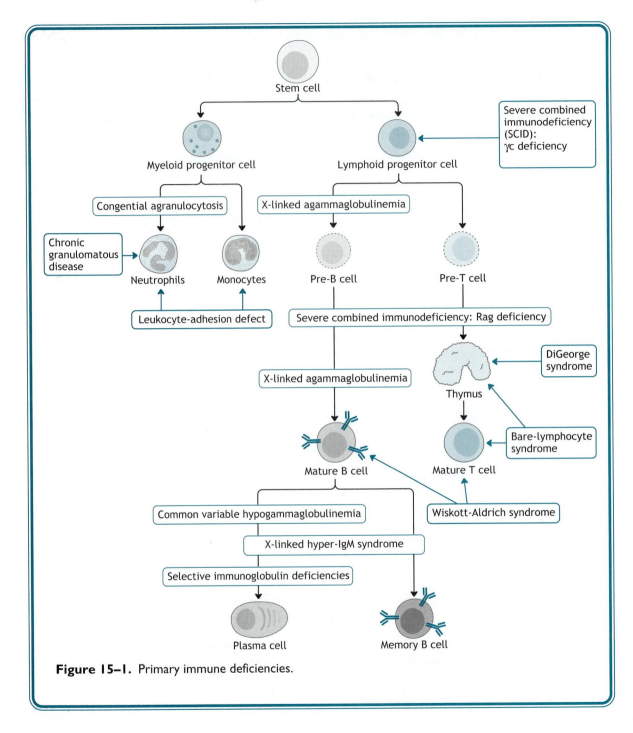

Figure 15–1. Primary immune deficiencies.

Table 15–1. Examples of selective primary T and B cell deficiencies.[a]

Category of Deficiency	Examples	Molecular or Cellular Defect	Clinical Presentation	Therapies
Antibody or humoral immunity	XID	Btk kinase mutation	Infections with extracellular bacteria commencing at 6–9 months of age	Antibiotics, IVIG
	Selective IgA deficiency	Varied	Sinopulmonary infections and diarrhea; increased incidence of atopic allergies	Antibiotics
	Hyper-IgM syndrome	CD154 or AID mutations	Elevated IgM; little or no IgG or IgA; absence of Ig class switching; bacterial infections	Antibiotics, IVIG
T cell or cellular immunity	DiGeorge syndrome	Thymic epithelium	Parathyroid deficiency; heart defects; early onset of fungal and viral infections; lymphopenia	Antimicrobial agents; thymic transplant
	BLS-II	Transcription of HLA class II genes	Absence of HLA-D expression; opportunistic viral and fungal infections; CD4$^+$ T cell lymphopenia	Antimicrobial agents; stem cell transplant
	Deficiency of TCR signaling	ZAP-70 mutation	Recurrent viral and fungal infections; depressed cellular immunity	Antimicrobial agents; stem cell transplant

[a]XID, X-linked immunodeficiency; Btk, Bruton's tyrosine kinase; Ig, immunoglobulin; IVIG, intravenous immunoglobulin; AID, activation-induced cytidine deaminase; BLS-II, bare lymphocyte syndrome type II; TCR, T cell receptor; ZAP-70, ζ-associated protein-70.

3. Conversely, the successful resolution of an infection aids in establishing a differential diagnosis of immune deficiency diseases.
   a. Children who resolve a viral infection (eg, chickenpox) in a normal manner are not likely to be deficient in T cells.
   b. Patients who do not have a history of recurrent bacterial infections probably have normal neutrophil function.

4. The nature of the infectious agent can suggest the type of selective immune deficiency.
   a. Patients with primary antibody, phagocytic cell, or complement deficiencies present with recurrent infections involving **extracellular bacteria** and certain **fungi**.
   b. Patients with primary T cell or combined [T cell plus antibody and/or natural killer (NK) cell] immune deficiencies present with recurrent infections involving **viruses, intracellular bacteria, fungi,** and certain **parasites**.

C. A differential diagnosis is essential for determining appropriate therapy.
   1. Antibody, phagocytic cell, and complement deficiencies present with similar types of infections, but require distinct therapies.
   2. Similarly, deficiencies in recombination activating gene 1 (Rag1), transporter associated with antigen processing (TAP)-1, and thymus development present with similar opportunistic virus infections.

II. Antibody deficiencies are the most common immune deficiency state in infants and children, accounting for nearly half of all conditions (Table 15–2).

A. The prevalence of these diseases ranges from a few reported cases to 1 case per 350 individuals.

B. Antibody deficiencies range from generalized **agammaglobulinemia** to selective immunoglobulin (Ig) (sub)class deficiencies (eg, IgG_2 deficiency).

C. Some patients with normal serum levels of Igs fail to make antibodies to important microbial antigens.

D. The most frequent antibody deficiencies represent a failure to synthesize or secrete Ig, rather than an absence of B cells.
   1. **Selective IgA deficiency** is the most common primary immune deficiency with a frequency of 1 in 350.
      a. In some patients, IgA is synthesized but not secreted.

Table 15–2. Distinguishing features of primary antibody deficiencies.[a]

Disease	Distinguishing Features
Selective IgA deficiency	Most common primary immune deficiency; many affected individuals are asymptomatic; IVIG contraindicated
Selective IgG_2 deficiency	Impaired antibody responses to bacterial polysaccharide antigens; recurrent infections with encapsulated bacteria
Transient hypogamma-globulinemia of infancy	Delayed onset of IgM and IgG production; IVIG contraindicated; recurrent sinopulmonary infections
XLA	Absence of peripheral $CD19^+$ B cells; delayed onset to 6 months of age; X-linked; pyogenic bacterial infections

[a]Ig, immunoglobulin; IVIG, intravenous immunoglobulin; XLA, X-linked agammaglobulinemia.

b. Nearly half of IgA-deficient patients are asymptomatic due to the translocation of IgM across the mucosal epithelium.

  2. Selective IgG$_2$ deficiency is a common form of IgG deficiency.

      a. These patients do not respond to polysaccharide vaccines.

      b. Infections with encapsulated bacteria are common.

  3. Transient hypogammaglobulinemia of infancy is a condition that can lead
to infections toward the end of the first year of life.

      a. These infants have normal numbers of mature B cells.

      b. They show delayed IgG secretion that becomes apparent as maternal IgG
levels subside (ie, at 6–8 months of age).

      c. Otitis media, pneumonia, and diarrhea are common.

E. B cells are absent in only a few antibody deficiency diseases.

  1. X-linked agammaglobulinemia (XLA) is a mutation in the gene for Bruton's
tyrosine kinase (**Btk**).

      a. B cell development is blocked at the pre-B cell stage.

      b. XLA patients have a peripheral phenotype of $T^+B^-NK^+$.

      c. Normal levels of serum IgG are present at birth and wane over time.

      d. XLA patients suffer from recurrent infections with pyogenic (pus-forming)
extracellular bacteria.

  2. A similar phenotype is seen in patients with **Ig H chain locus deletions** that
prevent the expression of a functional μ chain.

  3. Igα deficiency blocks B cell development at the pre-B stage.

  4. κ-chain deficiency blocks the differentiation of κ-bearing B cells.

F. Most antibody deficiencies can be diagnosed using simple laboratory tests.

  1. Except for certain rare conditions (eg, XLA), the measurement of B cell numbers is not essential to establishing a diagnosis.

  2. Ig concentrations can be measured by nephelometry (Chapter 5).

  3. Isohemagglutinin titers reflect the ability to produce antibody.

  4. Responses to the tetanus toxoid and pneumococcal polysaccharide vaccines
provide information on memory and naive B cell function.

  5. A differential diagnosis requires the elimination of phagocytic cell and complement deficiencies.

G. The treatment of B cell deficiencies addresses both infections and the underlying
hypogammaglobulinemia.

  1. Antibiotics are given to treat bacterial infections.

  2. Intravenous immunoglobulins (IVIG) restore antibody levels.

      a. Because the half-life of IgG is approximately 3 weeks, IVIG must be given
frequently.

      b. IVIG is prepared from the pooled sera of immune donors.

      c. IVIG therapy is not recommended for children with transient hypogamma-
globulinemia of infancy or patients with selective IgA deficiency.

  3. Because IVIG is relatively safe and effective, stem cell transplantation is rarely
performed to correct B cell deficiencies.

IVIG AND SELECTIVE IGA DEFICIENCY

- *Selective IgA deficiency is an important exception to the general use of IVIG to treat antibody deficiencies.*

- *The use of IVIG in these patients carries a risk of anaphylactic or anaphylactoid shock.*

- *This is thought to result from the tendency of these patients to produce IgE and IgG antibodies to IgA that is present in the IVIG preparations.*
- *Such antibodies mediate type I and type III hypersensitivity responses to IVIG.*

III. Patients with primary T cell (T⁻B⁺NK⁺) and combined (T⁻B⁻NK⁺, T⁻ B⁺NK⁻, or T⁻B⁻NK⁻) immune deficiencies acquire infections in their first few weeks of life.

    A. These infections are **pediatric emergencies**.

        1. The infectious agents include **viruses, fungi,** and other **intracellular pathogens**.

        2. Many of the organisms that infect T cell-deficient patients (eg, *Cryptosporidium, Pneumocystis, Leishmania* species) show low virulence and only rarely cause disease in the general population.

        3. The infections in T cell-deficient patients are often disseminated and rapidly progressing.

GRAFT-VERSUS-HOST DISEASE (GVHD) IN PREGNANCY

- **GVHD** *is typically seen only in stem cell transplantation (Chapter 17).*
- *T cells of the donor recognize and attack the recipient's tissues.*
- *Because pregnancy provides an opportunity for maternal T cells to recognize fetal HLA antigens inherited from the father, GVHD can also occur in this setting.*
- *Because the fetal immune system is sufficiently mature to destroy maternal T cells that cross the placenta, the disease is rarely seen in normal pregnancies.*
- *However, when fetuses have congenital T cell deficiencies, GVHD can occur.*
- *GVHD also occurs when fresh whole blood is transfused to a T cell-deficient child.*

    B. Selective T cell deficiencies are due to blocks in thymocyte differentiation and/or receptor-initiated cell signaling (Table 15–3).

        1. DiGeorge syndrome is a rare thymic hypoplasia due to dysmorphogenesis of the third and fourth pharyngeal pouches.

            a. Embryonic abnormalities are also seen in the heart, major vessels, parathyroid, and facial structures.

            b. Antibody deficiency results from the absence of Th cells.

            c. T cell lymphopenia and opportunisitic viral and fungal (eg, *Pneumocystis*) infections result.

        2. Defects in **T cell receptor (TCR)-initiated signaling** (Chapter 6) cause deficiencies in cell-mediated immunity.

            a. Loss-of-function mutations exist in **CD3ζ, Lck,** and **ζ-associated protein-70 (ZAP-70)**.

            b. Defective positive selection in the thymus causes peripheral lymphopenia with a **T⁻B⁺NK⁺** phenotype.

        3. Bare lymphocyte syndrome type I (BLS-I) is a selective deficiency of CD8⁺ T cells.

            a. This condition is caused by mutations in the **TAP** proteins.

            b. Major histocompatibility complex (MHC) class I expression and positive selection in the thymus are impaired.

            c. The peripheral lymphocyte phenotype is **CD4⁺CD8⁻B⁺NK⁺.**

Table 15–3. Distinguishing features of primary T cell deficiencies.[a]

Disease	Distinguishing Features
DiGeorge syndrome	Lymphopenia with hypoparathyroidism, cardiac and facial defects; corrected by thymic transplant
ZAP-70 or CD3ζ deficiency	Absence of both CD4$^+$ and CD8$^+$ T cell function with normal numbers of B cells and NK cells
BLS type I	Absence of HLA class I expression and decreased numbers of CD8$^+$ T cells
BLS type II	Absence of HLA class II expression and decreased numbers of CD4$^+$ T cells
Th1 deficiency	Decreased IL-12 and IFN-γ signaling; mycobacterial pneumonia
Hyper-IgM syndrome type I	Absence of CD154; elevated IgM antibody responses; decreased IgG and IgA
AID deficiency	Elevated IgM antibody responses; normal expression of CD154 and CD40

[a]ZAP-70, ζ-associated protein-70; NK, natural killer; BLS, bare lymphocyte syndrome; IL, interleukin; IFN, interferon; Ig, immunoglobulin; AID, activation-induced cytidine deaminase.

4. **Bare lymphocyte syndrome type II (BLS-II)** results in a **CD4$^-$CD8$^+$B$^+$NK$^+$** phenotype.
   a. These patients have mutations in transcription factors, such as **CIITA**, that coordinately regulate MHC class II gene expression.
   b. Positive selection of CD4$^+$ thymocytes is impaired.
   c. The activation of peripheral CD4$^+$ T cells is blocked.
5. A family of related **Th 1 cell deficiencies** is caused by deficient cytokine signaling.
   a. **Interleukin (IL)-12** and **IL-12 receptor** defects block Th1 cell differentiation and activation.
   b. **Interferon (IFN)-γ receptor deficiency** blocks macrophage activation.
   c. Recurrent infections with intracellular bacteria (eg, *Mycobacterium* and *Salmonella* species) result.
6. The absence of the coreceptor CD40 or its ligand, CD154, causes **hyper-IgM syndrome type 1**.
   a. This leads to a deficiency of the Th2 signals necessary for Ig class switching in B cells (Chapter 6).
   b. Patients have elevated levels of IgM antibodies, but no IgG, IgA, or IgE.
7. **Hyper-IgM syndrome type 2** results from a mutation in the gene for **activation-induced cytidine deaminase (AID)** (Chapter 9).

a. T helper cell signaling for Ig class switching is absent.

    b. Somatic hypermutation and affinity maturation in B cells are also impaired.

C. Severe combined immune deficiency (SCID) is caused by a number of different genetic mutations (Table 15–4).

    1. The X-linked recessive form of SCID is most prevalent.

        a. It is caused by an absence of the **common γ chain (γc)** of the receptors for IL-2, IL-4, IL-7, IL-9, and IL-15.

        b. Abnormal development of T cells and NK cells results in a **T$^-$B$^+$NK$^-$** phenotype.

    2. The same phenotype (**T$^-$B$^+$NK$^-$**) is seen in deficiencies of **Janus kinase 3 (Jak3)**, which mediates signaling from these receptors.

    3. Mutations in the gene coding for the enzyme **adenosine deaminase (ADA)** cause SCID.

        a. ADA catalyzes the breakdown of intracellular adenosine and deoxyadenosine.

        b. Excess adenosine inhibits methyltransferase reactions in T cells, B cells, and NK cells resulting in a **T$^-$B$^-$NK$^-$** phenotype.

    4. Mutations in the **Rag1** and **recombination activating gene 2 (Rag2)** genes block T and B cell development by preventing TCR and B cell receptor (BCR) gene rearrangements.

        a. Lymphocyte differentiation is blocked at the pre-T and pre-B cell stages.

        b. The lymphocyte phenotype in this condition is **T$^-$B$^-$NK$^+$.**

    5. Wiscott–Aldrich syndrome (WAS) is a condition characterized by thrombocytopenia and immune deficiency.

    6. Perforin and granzyme deficiencies manifest as decreased T cell and NK cell cytotoxic activity.

Table 15–4. Distinguishing features of primary SCID.[a]

Gene Mutation	Overall Cellular Phenotype	Distinguishing Features
γc	T$^-$B$^+$NK$^-$	Most frequent cause; impaired signaling through multiple cytokine receptors; normal B cell numbers
Jak3	T$^-$B$^+$NK$^-$	Rare, but otherwise indistinguishable from γc deficiency
ADA	T$^-$B$^-$NK$^-$	Decline in the numbers of all lymphocyte subsets over time
Rag1, Rag2	T$^-$B$^-$NK$^+$	Absence of peripheral T and B cells from birth; normal NK cells

[a]Jak3, Janus kinase 3; ADA, adenosine deaminase; Rag1, Rag2, recombination activating genes 1 and 2; NK, natural killer.

D. The **diagnosis** of T cell and combined immune deficiencies depends on recognizing the typical infections that characterize these conditions and measuring lymphocyte numbers and functions.

1. Infections begin in the first few months of life.
2. Lymphopenia is common.
3. Measuring anti-HIV antibodies or viral load is essential when a T cell deficiency is suspected.
4. Measuring CD3, CD4, CD8, CD19, and CD154 expression by flow cytometry can help detect lymphocyte subset deficiencies.
5. T cell proliferation in response to polyclonal activators (the plant mitogen phytohemagglutinin) can be measured in vitro.
6. Delayed-type hypersensitivity (DTH) skin tests (eg, intradermal or patch testing) are used to evaluate CD4$^+$ Th1 cell responses to common microbes.

E. **Therapy** includes antiviral and antifungal agents and hematopoietic stem cell replacement.

1. **Thymus transplantation** is effective in treating DiGeorge syndrome.
2. **Stem cell transplantation** (Chapter 17) is effective for SCID and selective T cell deficiency patients.
3. **Gene therapy** is being tested for some of these immune deficiencies (eg, ADA deficiency).
4. Other therapies are **contraindicated**.
   a. T cell-deficient patients should not be immunized with **live viral vaccines**.
   b. All blood products (whole blood, platelets, and plasma) should be irradiated prior to transfusion.

GENE THERAPY FOR IMMUNE DEFICIENCIES

- *The identification of specific genetic mutations that cause immunodeficiency diseases provides the opportunity to correct these conditions by gene therapy.*
- *The most promising approach appears to be "repairing" the defective gene within the patient's own hematopoietic stem cells by retroviral transfer followed by reinfusion.*
- *ADA deficiency was the first human disease treated by gene therapy in the 1990s.*
- *Other immune deficiencies that have been considered include γc deficiency, leukocyte adhesion defect (LAD; CD18 deficiency), and chronic granulomatous disease (respiratory burst deficiency).*

IV. Primary **phagocytic cell deficiencies** result from decreased cell number, abnormal cell adhesion and migration, defective intracellular granules, or impaired intracellular killing mechanisms (Table 15–5).

A. **Cyclic neutropenia** is caused by a mutation in the **neutrophil elastase** gene.
   1. Neutropenia (< 200 cells/μL) occurs periodically.
   2. Treatment with recombinant **colony-stimulating factor-granulocyte (CSF-G)** has proven effective.

B. **LAD** is characterized by poor leukocyte adhesion to the vascular endothelium, delayed wound healing, and defective complement-dependent opsonophagocytosis.
   1. **LAD type 1** is a mutation in the gene for **CD18**, a β2 integrin family member (Chapter 8).
      a. Patients show chronic leukocytosis involving neutrophils and fail to phagocytize iC3b-coated particles.

Table 15–5. Distinguishing features of phagocytic cell deficiencies.[a]

Disease	Distinguishing Features
Cyclic neutropenia	Oscillating neutropenia; responsiveness to CSF-G
LAD type 1	Chronic leukocytosis; absence of CD18-containing receptors; limited neutrophil extravasation and pus formation; impaired iC3b-mediated phagocytosis
LAD type 2	Leukocytosis; infections; normal CD18
LAD type 3	Decreased selectin expression
LAD type 4	Impaired CD18 initiated signaling
Chediak–Higashi syndrome	Formation of giant fused granules in neutrophils and NK cells
CGD	Absence of superoxide production; infections with catalase-positive microbes; granulomas
Job's syndrome	Decreased IFN-γ synthesis; IgE levels, skin abscesses without erythema or tenderness
Th1 pathway defects	Impaired macrophage activation

[a]CSF-G, colony-stimulating factor-granulocyte; IFN, interferon; LAD, leukocyte adhesion defect; NK, natural killer; CGD, chronic granulomatous disease.

    b. Diagnosis is aided by demonstrating the absence of CD11 or CD18 on blood leukocytes.
   2. LAD type 2 is a defect in fucose metabolism that impairs selectin function.
   3. LAD type 3 is a defect in selectin expression.
   4. LAD type 4 is caused by a mutation in the rac signaling molecule activated by CD18.
  C. Chediak–Higashi syndrome (CHS) results from the excessive fusion of granules in a number of granulated cells, including leukocytes.
    1. The defect is caused by a mutation in a regulator of lysosomal trafficking.
    2. CHS cells show poor chemotaxis and impaired NK cell function.
  D. Neutrophil-specific granule deficiencies, including the absence of α and β defensins, result in impaired intracellular killing of microbes.

IMMUNE DEFICIENCY IN JOB'S SYNDROME

- *Job's syndrome* (hyper-IgE syndrome; Chapter 13) is characterized by highly elevated levels of serum IgE, eczema, and sinopulmonary and skin infections.
- Given the elevated IgE levels, atopic dermatitis is a common misdiagnosis.
- Infections can cause deep skin and lung abscesses.

- *An unusual characteristic of the skin lesions is the absence of erythema, tenderness, and warmth, similar to the appearance of the skin boils of the biblical character Job.*
- *A marked decrease of IFN-γ production by these patients may explain both the elevated IgE levels and the impaired phagocyte responses to infection.*

    E. Chronic granulomatous disease (CGD) is a heterogeneous condition caused by a defective respiratory burst oxidase.
        1. Mutations in any of four subunit genes have been reported.
        2. Diagnosis is based on the nitroblue tetrazolium (NBT) dye reduction test for oxidant production.
        3. CGD is characterized by bacterial and fungal infections, especially *Staphylococcus* and *Aspergillus* species.
        4. Granulomas form in the lungs, liver, and spleen when microbes that cannot be killed are "walled off."
        5. Prophylactic antibiotics, recombinant IFN-γ, and granulocyte transfusions are beneficial.
        6. Stem cell transplantation is potentially curative.
    F. Myeloperoxidase (MPO) deficiency causes a block in the production of hypohalous acids.
    G. Aggressive **treatment** with antibiotics is necessary to control infections in phagocytic cell deficiencies.
        1. Some conditions benefit from prophylactic antimicrobial agents.
        2. Recombinant cytokines are of value in treating cyclic neutropenia and CGD.
        3. Leukocyte transfusions during acute infections are beneficial.
        4. Stem cell transplantation is potentially curative in CGD, Chediak–Higashi syndrome, and LAD.

ANTIBIOTICS AND PHAGOCYTE DEFICIENCIES

- *Neutrophil deficiencies tend to manifest as gingivitis and periodontal diseases, cutaneous infections and abscesses, pneumonias, and/or granulomas caused by multiple infectious agents.*
- *While IFN-γ deficiency affects macrophage function and results in infections primarily with intracellular bacterial pathogens, diverse types of pathogens cause infections in Chediak–Higashi syndrome or cyclic neutropenia.*
- *Prophylactic antimicrobial therapy is less effective when infections are caused by diverse microbial species.*

    V. Inherited deficiencies in the **complement system** cause both infectious and noninfectious diseases (Table 15–6).
    A. Rare deficiencies in all of the individual components have been described.
        1. A deficiency of **mannose-binding protein (MBP)** is the most common single component defect.
        2. C2 deficiency is the most common deficiency affecting the classical pathway.
    B. Deficiencies in the classical, lectin, or alternative pathways can increase the susceptibility to bacterial and some viral infections.
        1. Early pathway deficiencies result in recurrent pyogenic infections.
        2. Defects in the terminal components C5–C8 lead to disseminated *Neisseria* infections.

Table 15–6. Primary deficiencies in the complement system.

Type of Deficiency	Components Involved	Clinical Characteristics
Classical pathway	C1q,r,s, C4, C2	Lupus nephritis Bacterial, viral, and fungal infections
Alternative pathway	P, B, D	*Neisseria* infections Pyogenic infections
Lectin pathway	MBL	Diverse infections
Common components	C3	Pyogenic infections
Terminal components	C5–C8	Disseminated *Neisseria* infections
Inhibitors	C1 Inh, H, I, C4b-BP	Angioedema, nephritis, infections
Cell surface inhibitors	DAF, CD59	Paroxysmal nocturnal hemoglobinuria
Receptors	CR3, CR4	Leukocyte adhesion, pyogenic infections, delayed wound healing

C. Defects in the expression of the **complement regulatory components** cause both infectious and noninfectious diseases.
1. **Factor I deficiency** increases the risk of pyogenic infections, including meningococcal meningitis.
   a. Unrestrained complement activation leads to C3 consumption (Chapter 8).
   b. Exogenous Factor I provides relief in acute disease.
2. **Factor H deficiency** also results in increased complement activation, C3 depletion, and an increased risk of infection.
3. **C1 inhibitor (C1 Inh) deficiency (hereditary angioedema)** and **C4b-BP deficiency** are characterized by episodic cutaneous and submucosal edema.
   a. Both conditions result in unabated activation of the classical complement pathway.
   b. A C2-derived peptide is thought to cause increased vascular permeability and localized edema in hereditary angioedema.
   c. C1 Inh also regulates the production of bradykinin, which can have a similar effect on endothelial permeability.
4. **Paroxysmal nocturnal hemoglobinuria (PNH)** is due to a failure of cells to express glycosylphosphatidylinositol (GPI)-linked membrane proteins, including CD59 and CD55 (decay accelerating factor).
   a. CD59 blocks insertion of C8 and C9 into the membrane.
   b. CD55 inhibits C3 and C5 convertases on the cell surface.
   c. Erythrocytes of PNH patients are highly susceptible to complement-mediated lysis.

D. Complement deficiencies and **autoimmunity** are often associated with one another.

    1. Patients with defects in the early classical pathway components often develop a lupus-like nephritis.

    2. Circulating immune complexes in autoimmunity deplete the early classical components.

    3. Autoantibodies to complement components (eg, anti-C1q) are sometimes produced by patients with systemic lupus erythematosus (SLE) (Chapter 16).

    4. Patients with SLE, Sjögren's syndrome, and autoimmune hemolytic anemias often show decreased expression of **complement receptor 1 (CR1)** on their erythrocytes.

E. The treatment of complement deficiencies focuses primarily on controlling infections and correcting acute symptoms.

    1. Aggressive antibiotic therapy is the first objective for infections.

    2. Plasma infusion or injection of individual components (eg, recombinant C1 Inh) has some clinical value for acute disease.

    3. The various treatments for autoimmunity associated with complement deficiencies are discussed in Chapter 17.

VI. Inherited innate immune defects can cause inflammatory or infectious diseases.

    A. An increased susceptibility to infections results from mutations in **interleukin-1 receptor-associated kinase (IRAK)** of the Toll-like receptors.

    B. Mutations in **mannose-binding lectin** increase the risk of infection, especially in the presence of other chronic diseases (eg, cystic fibrosis).

    C. Deficiencies in the antimicrobial **Nod proteins** (Chapter 1) are thought to contribute to the induction of inflammatory bowel disease.

VII. Acquired or secondary immune deficiency states typically show adult onset.

    A. Acquired immune deficiencies can also result from **infections**.

        1. Acquired immune deficiency syndrome (AIDS) is the most prevalent immune deficiency in the United States.

            a. $CD4^+$ T cells are depleted by the lymphotrophic virus **human immunodeficiency virus-1 (HIV-1)**.

            b. Th1 cell functions are particularly affected.

            c. Opportunistic infections with intracellular pathogens (Table 15–7) are the primary causes of morbidity and mortality.

        2. Transient neutropenia in children is seen in some viral (eg, measles) and bacterial (eg, tuberculosis) infections.

        3. A number of microbial pathogens (eg, herpesviruses) have developed immune evasion mechanisms that cause selective immunosuppression of the host (Chapter 14).

    B. Immune deficiency can arise secondary to **therapy**.

        1. Splenectomy impairs the ability to produce antibodies.

            a. Splenectomized patients are at increased risk for sepsis.

            b. Splenectomy decreases IgG antibody responses to polysaccharide vaccines.

        2. Immunosuppressive drugs increase the risk of infections.

Table 15–7. Opportunistic pathogens causing infections in AIDS.

Bacteria	Fungi	Viruses	Parasites
Mycobacteria	*Pneumocystis*	Herpes simplex	*Toxoplasma*
Salmonella	*Cryptococcus*	Cytomegalovirus	*Cryptosporidium*
	Candida	Varicella-Zoster	*Leishmania*

     a. Many **chemotherapeutic agents** used to treat malignancies are immunosuppressive.

     b. Drugs that block allograft rejection (Chapter 17) also inhibit immune responses to microbial pathogens.

     c. **Corticosteroids** increase the risk of infection when used at high doses or over long periods of time.

     d. **Disease-modifying antirheumatic drugs (DMARDS)** used for treating chronic autoimmune diseases carry a similar risk of increasing infection rates.

     e. The use of certain **anticytokine reagents** can inhibit protective immunity to specific pathogens [eg, antitumor necrosis factor (TNF)-α antibodies and tuberculosis].

  C. **Cancer** is a common cause of secondary immune deficiencies.

     1. Malignancies that grow within the bone suppress hematopoiesis, including lymphopoiesis and granulopoiesis.

     2. Lymphoid malignancies (eg, lymphomas) inhibit normal lymphocyte functions in the peripheral lymphoid tissues.

     3. Cancer cells often produce excessive quantities of cytokines and growth factors that cause immune imbalance.

  D. **Protein-losing enteropathies, extensive burns**, and **nephrotic syndrome** result in protein loss, hypogammaglobulinemia, and hypocomplementemia.

  E. **Common variable immune deficiency** is a heterogeneous syndrome that shows early or adult onset.

     1. B cell numbers are normal, but plasma cells are infrequent and antibody production is impaired.

     2. T cell numbers and subsets are also typically normal, but cellular immunity can be decreased.

     3. Bacterial agents constitute the greatest threats of infection, which resemble those seen in XLA.

CLINICAL PROBLEMS

A 4-year-old child is referred with the diagnosis of type 1 LAD. She has a history of recurrent bacterial infections, including pneumonias and skin abscesses. Radiography demonstrates granuloma-like lesions in her lungs and liver. However, the data in the following table suggest this condition has not been properly diagnosed.

1. Which of the elements in the table is **inconsistent** with a diagnosis of type 1 LAD?

CD Marker	Patient (%)	Normal Range (%)
CD2	76	75–92
CD3	75	60–85
CD4	52	30–65
CD8	26	20–52
CD11a	65	65–85
CD18	73	70–86
CD19	12	7–17
CD45	52	44–62

    A. The CD2 value

    B. The CD19 value

    C. The CD11a value

    D. The CD45 value

    E. The CD3 value

A 3-month-old child presents with a history of persistent diarrhea and oral thrush beginning at age 3 weeks and has developed signs and symptoms consistent with *Pneumocystis carinii* pneumonia. Both he and his parents are HIV negative based on serological and polymerase chain reaction (PCR) testing. Complete blood counts demonstrate profound lymphopenia.

2. Which of the following blood cell types should show normal numbers if this condition was caused by a Rag deficiency?

    A. CD3$^+$ cells with a CD4 coreceptor

    B. CD19$^+$ cells

    C. Single-positive thymocytes

    D. Memory B cells

    E. NK cells

An 8-month-old male child has an apparent antibody deficiency. The diagnosis has been narrowed to two possibilities.

3. Measuring which of the following immune parameters would distinguish hyper-IgM syndrome (type 1) from X-linked agammaglobulinemia?

    A. IgG levels in the serum

    B. CD19$^+$ cells in the blood

    C. IL-2 production by the patient's lymphocytes in vitro

D. NK cell-mediated cytotoxicity in vitro

E. IgA levels in the saliva

A pediatric patient has a history of recurrent infections, and it is hypothesized that she has a defect in the neutrophil-mediated killing of phagocytized bacteria.

4. Which of the following laboratory assays would most directly test this hypothesis?

A. Complement fixation test

B. Quantitative test for serum Igs

C. NBT dye reduction test

D. Flow cytometry for CD18 expression

E. Complete blood count and differential

An adolescent with a history of childhood upper respiratory tract infections and diarrhea continues to have recurring sinusitis, which is attributed to *Pseudomonas aeruginosa*, a gram-negative bacterium. Laboratory tests over the past 5 years have repeatedly indicated that he has normal T cell numbers (based on CD3, CD4, and CD8), normal serum complement levels and activity, and normal serum IgM and IgG levels for his age. Isohemagglutinin titers are normal. Neutrophil numbers and function (chemotaxis, opsonophagocytosis, and respiratory burst) are all normal. His IgG antibody response to tetanus toxoid challenge is also within the normal range. He shows 4+ reactions in delayed hypersensitivity skin tests against several common fungal antigens.

5. What therapy is appropriate for this patient?

A. Antibiotics only

B. Antibiotics and IVIG

C. Antibiotics, IVIG, and stem cell transplantation

D. Stem cell transplantation

E. Antibiotics and IFN-γ

Johnny is an 8-month-old child with recurrent fungal and viral infections. His blood lymphocyte numbers are normal and they bind IL-2 in vitro. It has been determined that his parents are both heterozygous for a mutation in their ZAP-70 genes that can explain Johnny's disease.

6. In addition to antimicrobial agents to treat his infections, what therapy should be considered for Johnny?

A. Thymus transplant

B. IVIG and all of the pediatric vaccines

C. Recombinant IL-2

D. Stem cell transplantation

E. Besides antimicrobial agents, there is no effective therapy for this patient.

ANSWERS

1. The correct answer is C. The diagnosis of LAD type 1 requires demonstrating that the patient lacks CD18 or any of the α chains that pair with the CD18 β chain (ie, CD11a, CD11b, or CD11c). This patient has normal levels of CD11a, which means she does not have LAD type 1.

2. The correct answer is E. Rag-deficient SCID patients show a $T^-B^-NK^+$ overall lymphocyte phenotype.

3. The correct answer is B. In hyper-IgM syndrome, normal numbers of B cells are present in the periphery. However, they do not receive the normal signaling from Th cells due to a defect in the coreceptor ligand CD154. In XLA the absence of the Btk kinase blocks B cell differentiation at the pre-B cell stage, and the patients have no peripheral $CD19^+$ B cells.

4. The correct answer is C. The NBT dye reduction test measures cellular production of oxidants, which are important in the oxygen-dependent killing of microbes by neutrophils (Chapter 1). The other tests could confirm phagocyte dysfunction as well, but would not directly relate to intracellular killing function.

5. The correct answer is A. This patient lacks any clear evidence of an immune deficiency that would explain his recurrent bacterial infections. There is no rationale for stem cell transplantation, and there is no antibody defect that would suggest giving IVIG. Only conventional antibiotic therapy is indicated for the treatment of the infection.

6. The correct answer is D. ZAP-70 deficiency affects TCR-initiated signaling in his T cells. Replacing the defective T cells with normal T cell precursors would theoretically be of value here.

CHAPTER 16
AUTOTOLERANCE
AND AUTOIMMUNITY

I. **Tolerance is an acquired condition of specific unresponsiveness to an antigen.**

A. **Autotolerance** (unresponsiveness to self antigens) is established within B and T lymphocytes as they encounter self antigens during development.

1. Self tolerance is antigen specific and can be induced either in a primary lymphoid organ or in the periphery.

2. Autotolerance continues to be established throughout life, even after the thymus atrophies.

B. Three mechanisms contribute to the induction of tolerance.

1. **Clonal deletion** results in the apoptosis of specific B and T cell clones.

   a. Clonal deletion generally occurs among immature B and T cells through a process called **negative selection** (Chapters 9 and 10).

   b. Deletion requires antigen recognition by immature lymphocytes through their B cell receptor (BCR) or T cell receptor (TCR).

2. **Clonal anergy** is a form of unresponsiveness in lymphocytes caused by antigen recognition in the absence of essential stimulatory coreceptor signals.

   a. Antigen presentation by antigen-presenting cells (APCs) that lack the B7 ligand for the CD28 coreceptor induces **T cell anergy**.

   b. Antigen presentation by cells that engage the inhibitory cytotoxic T lymphocyte-associated protein 4 (CTLA-4) coreceptor can also induce T cell anergy.

3. Tolerance, including autotolerance, can also be mediated by active suppressor cells in the periphery.

   a. **Regulatory T cells** (Treg cells) mediate unresponsiveness to specific antigens.

   b. Treg cells are induced in both the thymus and the periphery by autoantigens.

   c. Suppression is generally mediated by the production of inhibitory cytokines, such as interleukin (IL)-10 and transforming growth factor (TGF)-β.

C. Autotolerance is established at two levels.

1. **Central tolerance** to self antigens is established during the differentiation of B and T cells in the bone marrow and thymus, respectively.

   a. Central tolerance results in the deletion of autoreactive clones (negative selection).

    b. Self-specific B cells can be rescued from clonal deletion by undergoing secondary immunoglobulin (Ig) locus rearrangements (BCR editing.)

  2. **Peripheral tolerance** involves all three mechanisms of tolerance induction—deletion, anergy, and suppression.

    a. The induction of autotolerance in the periphery continues throughout life.

    b. Because quiescent autoreactive B and T cell clones reside in normal individuals, autoimmunity is common.

TRANSPLANTATION TOLERANCE

CLINICAL CORRELATION

- *It is not uncommon for transplant recipients to become tolerant to their foreign organ grafts over time, despite significant genetic disparities with the organ donor.*

- *Pretransplantation lymphoablation appears to favor the induction of tolerance, as does the establishment of donor–recipient chimerism when donor bone marrow cells are provided.*

- *The continual exposure of the recipient to the HLA antigens of the donor may also induce active suppressor cells, including Treg cells.*

- *Blocking CD28/B7 and CD40/CD154 costimulatory signaling may be another mechanism for inducing specific unresponsiveness to allografts.*

- *The ultimate goal of inducing transplantation tolerance is to reduce the dependence on powerful immunosuppressive therapies in the posttransplant period.*

II. Autoimmunity results from the loss of self tolerance.

  A. The **molecular mimicry theory of autoimmunity** proposes that autoimmunity occurs when microbial antigens cross-react with self antigens.

    1. Antibodies to the M protein of *Streptococcus pyogenes* that are induced during infection can react with cardiac autoantigens of the sarcolemma and heart valves and cause **rheumatic fever**.

    2. Antibodies to *Treponema pallidum* induced during syphilis can cross-react with human fibronectin and collagen.

    3. Antibodies to the insulin receptor are induced during papilloma virus infections.

  B. The **costimulatory theory of autoimmunity** proposes that silent autospecific lymphocytes are activated when tissues inappropriately express stimulatory coreceptor ligands.

    1. Major histocompatibility complex (MHC) class II molecules are expressed by pancreatic β cells in type 1 diabetes mellitus.

    2. Microglial cells of patients with multiple sclerosis express B7.

  C. Autoimmunity is induced when cryptic or **sequestered autoantigens** that are normally not seen by the immune system are released to the periphery.

    1. Autoimmune uveitis is thought to develop when ocular antigens released from a damaged eye induce immune damage to the contralateral eye.

    2. Autoantigens of spermatogonia can be recognized as nonself if they are later released from the testes by vasectomy.

  D. **Modified self antigens** can induce autoimmune responses.

    1. Autoimmune hemolytic anemias result when drugs bind to erythrocyte surface proteins.

    2. Autoantibodies to the Fc domains of IgG molecules (**rheumatoid factors**) are often produced in **rheumatoid arthritis**.

VASECTOMY AND AUTOIMMUNE ORCHITIS

- *Vasectomy is the most common means by which men elect permanent sterilization for the purpose of contraception.*
- *Vasectomy does not halt spermatogenesis, and sperm can become accessible to the immune system following the procedure.*
- *Sperm-agglutinating antibodies develop in over 50% of vasectomized males.*
- *Epididymitis and orchitis mediated by autoantibodies occur at a rate of 5–6%.*

III. Autoimmunity often exists without overt autoimmune disease.

A. The elderly commonly produce low-affinity autoantibodies that do not cause disease.

B. Witebsky's postulates establish a set of criteria for designating a disease as autoimmune in nature.

   1. Autoantibodies or autoreactive T cells must be demonstrated in the patient.

   2. The autoantigen(s) must be identified.

   3. Immunizing a laboratory animal with the autoantigen must induce a comparable autoimmune response and autoimmune disease.

   4. The disease manifestations must be transferable to a naive recipient with autoantibody or autospecific T cells.

C. Several human diseases appear to satisfy Witebsky's postulates.

   1. Myelin-specific T cells of the type found in **multiple sclerosis** can transfer disease to laboratory rats and mice.

   2. The lesions found in **myasthenia gravis** can be duplicated in animals by the transfer of patient serum.

   3. Harrington's experiments with **idiopathic thrombocytopenia purpura** clearly identify this condition as an autoimmune disease.

WILLIAM HARRINGTON AND IDIOPATHIC THROMBOCYTOPENIA PURPURA

- *In 1951, a young hematologist named William Harrington was caring for a group of patients with bleeding disorders and low platelet counts.*
- *Dr. Harrington proposed that their thrombocytopenia was immune based.*
- *After injecting himself with the plasma of one of his patients, he developed severe, but transient thrombocytopenia.*
- *Because his megakaryocytes were spared destruction, he eventually recovered.*
- *This experiment firmly established that autoantibodies can cause human disease.*

D. The diagnosis of autoimmune diseases is aided by laboratory tests.

   1. Some tests detect **tissue-bound autoantibodies**.

      a. Antibodies to glomerular basement membrane antigens in **Goodpasture's disease** show a characteristic linear distribution in the kidney by immunofluorescence.

      b. By contrast, the "lumpy-bumpy" appearance of IgG in the glomerulus is typical of immune complex autoimmune diseases (eg, **systemic lupus erythematosus or SLE**).

   2. Many laboratory tests are designed to detect **circulating autoantibodies**.

      a. Antinuclear antibodies (ANA) are detected by immunofluorescence.

(1) The autoantigens include DNA, histones, and nucleolar proteins.

(2) These antibodies are seen in SLE, Sjögren's syndrome, and scleroderma.

b. Antineutrophil cytoplasmic antigen (ANCA) is characteristic of certain forms of autoimmune nephritis and vasculitis (eg, Wegener's granulomatosis).

c. Rheumatoid factor (RF) is common to rheumatoid arthritis and a number of other autoimmune diseases.

(1) RF is an autoantibody to the Fc region of IgG.

(2) RF is mostly IgM anti-IgG, but IgG and IgA autoantibodies have also been described.

d. The **Coombs test** detects IgG antibodies on erythrocytes and platelets.

(1) These antibodies can be specific for endogenous or exogenous (ie, haptenic) cell surface antigens.

(2) "Coombs-positive" is synonymous with immune-based when used to describe an anemia.

3. Tests that measure the serum concentrations of **complement** can be used to follow the status of autoimmune diseases.

a. Complement activity is often depressed during acute exacerbations of immune complex autoimmune diseases.

b. Measuring complement levels can be useful for monitoring the success of therapy.

IV. The spectrum of autoimmune diseases ranges from those that are organ specific to those that are essentially systemic in nature.

A. In **organ-specific autoimmune diseases** symptoms reflect the distribution of the target autoantigen(s).

1. Hashimoto's thyroiditis, pernicious anemia, and Addison's disease are examples of organ-specific autoimmune diseases.

2. The organ-specific disease manifestations of these conditions (eg, thyroid dysfunction) are important clues to their diagnosis.

B. Systemic autoimmune diseases (ie, the **rheumatological disorders**) typically involve the skin, kidneys, muscles, joints, and blood vessels.

1. Tissue damage is widely distributed.

2. Symptoms can reflect the deposition of soluble immune complexes, which is an important step in disease pathogenesis.

AUTOIMMUNE POLYENDOCRINE SYNDROME

- *Autoimmune polyendocrine syndrome (APS) type 1 is a rare condition caused by a mutation in the gene for the transcription factor autoimmune regulator (AIRE).*
- *Patients present with chronic mucocutaneous candidiasis, hypoparathyroidism, and/or adrenal insufficiency.*
- *AIRE is expressed in thymic epithelial cells and may control induction of self tolerance.*
- *Twenty percent of affected individuals develop type 1 diabetes mellitus.*

C. Tissue damage and symptoms in autoimmune diseases can change with time, because autoantibody responses become increasingly polyspecific.

1. The initial autoantibody is specific for a dominant self epitope.

2. Autoimmunity broadens with time by **epitope spreading** (Figure 16–1).

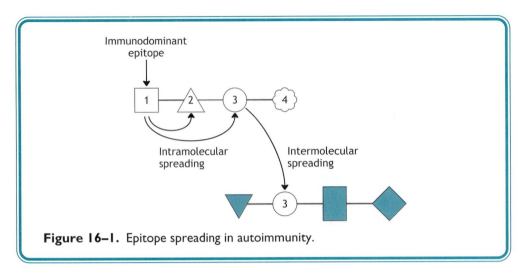

Figure 16–1. Epitope spreading in autoimmunity.

    a. B cells specific for the initial epitope elicit new responses by presenting additional epitopes on the same antigen (**intramolecular spreading**).

    b. B cells specific for the epitopes of the first autoantigen can cross-react with a second autoantigen (**intermolecular spreading**).

V. One of four pathogenic mechanisms underlies the development of most autoimmune diseases (Table 16–1).

  A. Antireceptor autoantibodies can cause autoimmune disease.

    1. Myasthenia gravis is a neurological condition presenting as muscle weakness and fatigue.

      a. Manifestations include diplopia, dysphonia, and difficulty swallowing, breathing, and walking.

      b. Antagonistic antibodies to the **acetylcholine receptor** block neurotransmission at motor end plates.

    2. Grave's disease is mediated by agonistic antibodies to the thyroid-stimulating hormone (TSH) receptor.

      a. Anti-TSH receptor antibodies are diagnostic.

      b. Hyperthyroidism and thyroid hyperplasia are common.

      c. Females are affected seven times more often than males.

      d. Many patients require thyroid ablation by radiotherapy or surgery.

  B. Cytotoxic immune tissue injury is the basis for many forms of organ-specific autoimmune disease.

    1. Coombs-positive hemolytic anemias and thrombocytopenias result from the immune lysis and/or clearance of blood cells.

      a. Complement plays a central role in cell destruction.

      b. "**Cold reactive antibodies**" are IgM and show high avidity.

        (1) They are more commonly found after certain infections (eg, mycoplasma).

        (2) They typically induce intravascular hemolysis.

      c. "**Warm reactive antibodies**" are IgG and have a lower avidity.

Table 16–1. Major pathogenic mechanisms underlying autoimmune diseases.

Mechanism of Disease	Examples	Initial Target Autoantigen	Distinguishing Clinical Features
Antireceptor autoantibody	Myasthenia gravis	Acetylcholine receptor	Muscle fatiguability
	Grave's disease	Thyroid-stimulating hormone receptor	Hyperthyroidism; goiter
	Pernicious anemia	Intrinsic factor	Vitamin B_{12} deficiency
	Addison's disease	Adrenal cell antigens	Adrenal insufficiency
Cytotoxic immune injury	Coombs-positive hemolytic anemia	Endogenous erythrocyte antigens or haptens	Intravascular hemolysis, clearance, and anemia
	Crohn's disease	Unknown	Transmural colitis and ileitis, ulceration
	Goodpasture's disease	Basement membrane collagen	Nephritis, pneumonitis
	Pemphigus vulgaris	Desmosome antigens in the skin	Blistering skin lesions, immunoglobulin G staining on epidermal cells
	Rheumatic fever	Cardiac muscle antigens	Heart valve damage
	Sjögren's syndrome	Nucleoproteins Ro and La	Dry eyes and mouth
	Thrombocytopenia purpura	Platelet integrins	Hemorrhagic purpura
Immune complex tissue injury	Drug-induced serum sickness	Drug hapten	Vasculitis, hemorrhage, arthralgia, nephritis
	Rheumatoid arthritis	Unknown	Synovitis, arthritis, cartilage and bone loss
	Systemic lupus erythematosus	Nucleic acids, nucleoproteins	Malar skin rash, arthralgia, anemia, arthritis, nephritis
Cellular immune tissue injury	Diabetes mellitus (type 1)	β cell antigens	Hyperglycemia; pancreatic β cell loss
	Hashimoto's thyroiditis	Thyroglobulin; thyroid peroxidase	Hypothyroidism
	Multiple sclerosis	Myelin proteins	Progressing sensory deficits, fatigue, weakness

(1) These antibodies cause Fc receptor-mediated clearance of erythrocytes.
(2) They are often induced by drugs that bind to cell surface proteins.
2. The **direct Coombs test** detects IgG antibodies on a patient's erythrocytes.
3. The **indirect Coombs test** detects circulating IgG autoantibodies that can react with endogenous erythrocyte antigens (eg, Rh).

4. **Drug-induced autoimmune hemolytic anemias** are caused by several mechanisms.
   a. Penicillin induces **direct Coombs-positive** anemias.
      (1) The drug binds directly to the erythrocyte surface and induces an antidrug antibody.
      (2) These conditions improve when the drug is discontinued.
   b. Methyldopa induces anemias that are **direct and indirect Coombs positive**.
      (1) This drug induces an antidrug antibody that cross-reacts with an Rh antigen.
      (2) Treatment may require immunosuppression and/or plasmapheresis to remove the autoantibodies.
   c. Other drugs can induce autoantibodies that form immune complexes with the drug.
      (1) The immune complexes can bind to the erythrocyte surface through CR1 (Chapter 8).
      (2) Such conditions are direct and indirect Coombs positive.
      (3) Treatment may require immunosuppression and/or plasmapheresis to remove the immune complexes.

5. **Goodpasture's disease** is mediated by IgG antibodies to basement membrane antigens, which together with neutrophils cause nephritis and pneumonitis.
   a. Autoantibodies in this disease are directed at epitopes of type IV collagen that are found in basement membranes.
   b. Treatment involves antiinflammatory and immunosuppressive drugs and plasmapheresis.
   c. End-stage renal disease may require kidney transplantation.

INFECTIONS AND AUTOIMMUNITY

- *An increased incidence of infection is not always seen in autoimmune diseases.*
- *However, when autoimmunity adversely affects the integrity of an epithelial barrier (eg, Crohn's disease or Sjögren's syndrome) opportunistic infections can occur.*
- *Complement consumption in immune complex autoimmune diseases can also impair host responses to infectious agents.*
- *Immunosuppressive therapies for autoimmunity increase the risks of infection.*
- *Paradoxically, with a decrease in the overall infection rate in developed countries, an increase in the incidence of allergy and autoimmune disease has occurred.*
- *This may reflect the failure of a microbe-poor environment to induce adequate inhibitory immune responses (eg, Treg cells) that prevent allergy and autoimmunity.*

C. **Immune complex-mediated diseases** share certain clinical features.
   1. **Drug-induced serum sickness** results when antibodies to drugs (eg, penicillin) form soluble immune complexes with their antigens.
      a. These complexes deposit in the skin, blood vessel walls, joints, and kidneys, activate complement, and recruit inflammatory cells.
      b. Vasculitis, hemorrhage, arthralgia, skin rashes, and nephritis are among the principal clinical findings.
   2. **SLE** is one of the most common autoimmune disease in women 20–40 years of age, especially African-Americans (Table 16–2).

Table 16–2. Epidemiology of autoimmune diseases.

Disease	HLA Associations	Female to Male Ratios	Approximate Incidence (per 100,000)
Myasthenia gravis	A1, B8, DR4		3
Grave's disease		7	100–300
Addison's disease	DR3, DR4		4
Sjögren's syndrome	B8, DRw52, DR3	9	<600
Crohn's disease	DR1 with DQw5		200
Pemphigus	DR4, DRw6		3
SLE[a]	DR2, DR3	5	50
Diabetes mellitus (type 1)	DR4 or DR1 with DQ1	<1	250
Rheumatoid arthritis	DR4, DR1	3	1000–3000
Hashimoto's thyroiditis	DR3, DR4, DR5	10	500

[a]SLE, systemic lupus erythematosus.

    a. The condition is characterized by fever, arthralgia, nonerosive arthritis, myalgia, photosensitivity, skin rashes, anemia, and glomerulonephritis.
    b. The autoantibodies produced in patients with SLE become increasingly polyspecific with epitope spreading.
        (1) Antibodies to **double-stranded DNA** are diagnostic.
        (2) Additional autoantibodies are produced against nuclear antigens (histones, ribonuclear proteins) and erythrocyte surface antigens.
    c. Immunofluorescence staining for immune complexes or C3b in the kidney shows a "lumpy-bumpy" pattern.
    d. Therapy for this condition is directed at reducing pain, inflammation, and autoantibody production (Table 16–3).
  3. Rheumatoid arthritis is the most common autoimmune disease in the United States today.
    a. Patients usually first present with morning stiffness and joint pain.
    b. Synovitis results from the infiltration of lymphocytes and macrophages and synovial growth in the form of a **pannus**.
    c. Th1 cells infiltrate the joint and contribute to macrophage and osteoclast activation.

Table 16–3. Therapies used to treat autoimmune diseases.[a]

Treatment	Intent	Diseases
Plasmapheresis	Reduce circulating autoantibodies and immune complexes	Grave's disease, hemolytic anemias, SLE
NSAIDs	Reduce pain and inflammation	Rheumatic diseases in general
Corticosteroids	Antiinflammatory effects	RA, SLE
Cytotoxic drugs (azathioprine)	Inhibit lymphocyte activation and proliferation	SLE
Anticytokine reagents	Block proinflammatory cytokine effects	Crohn's disease (TNF-α), RA, (IL-1β or TNF-α)
Corrective surgery	Removal or replacement of damaged tissues	Crohn's disease, Hashimoto's thyroiditis, RA
Transfusion and transplantation	Organ or tissue replacement	Hemolytic anemias, type I diabetes mellitus

[a]SLE, systemic lupus erythematosus; NSAIDs, nonsteroidal antiinflammatory drugs; RA, rheumatoid arthritis; TNF, tumor necrosis factor; IL, interleukin.

  d. Macrophages activate matrix metalloproteases and osteoclasts, which leads to cartilage and bone erosion.
  e. Immune complexes, including rheumatoid factor, are present in the joint spaces.
  f. Therapy includes immunosuppression, synovectomy, and joint replacement (Table 16–3).
 D. Cell-mediated autoimmune diseases do not require autoantibodies.
  1. Multiple sclerosis is a neurodegenerative condition resulting from central nervous system (CNS) demyelination by activated macrophages.
   a. Inflammation is initiated by CD4⁺ T cells specific for myelin autoantigens (myelin basic protein, myelin oligodendrocyte glycoprotein).
   b. Th1 cytokines recruit and activate T cells and macrophages.
   c. MHC class II and the B7 coreceptor ligand are induced on astrocytes and microglia.
  2. Type 1 (immune-mediated) diabetes mellitus involves the destruction of pancreatic islet β cells and hyperglycemia.
   a. Target autoantigens include the insulin receptor, β cell granule proteins, and insulin.
   b. Increased HLA-DR expression on β cells is common.

c. CD4$^+$ Th1 cells, CD8$^+$ T cells, and macrophages infiltrate the islets and induce β cell apoptosis.

      d. Insulin replacement by injection, pancreas transplantation, or islet cell transplantation is the preferred therapy.

   3. Sjögren's syndrome is a disease involving T cell-mediated damage to lacrimal and salivary glands that leads to dry eyes and dry mouth (sicca symptoms).

CLINICAL PROBLEMS

A patient recently diagnosed with SLE is experiencing significant symptoms of 3 weeks duration that include edema and skin rash. Her serum blood urea nitrogen (BUN) and creatinine levels are increased, and a biopsy of her kidney shows IgG and C3b at the glomerular basement membrane. Her serum complement levels are monitored over time.

1. Which of the following findings would be most consistent with a worsening clinical course?

   A. A decline in C9 levels

   B. A decline in C3 and C4 levels

   C. An increase in Factor P levels

   D. An increase in C1 inhibitor (C1 Inh) levels

   E. A decline in C7 levels

2. Of the following laboratory test findings, which would have been most useful in making the initial diagnosis of this disease?

   A. A positive ANA

   B. A positive cross-match

   C. Bence–Jones urinary proteins

   D. A positive mixed lymphocyte reaction

   E. Antibodies to myelin basic protein

Helen's physician has prescribed methyldopa for the treatment of her hypertension. She visits the outpatient medicine clinic several months later complaining of fatigue and has a noticeable pale color in the palms of her hands. Her hemoglobin is 9.5 g/dL (normal range = 13–15 g/dL).

3. What laboratory test should be ordered to determine if her anemia is due to an antibody?

   A. HLA typing

   B. Antithyroglobulin

   C. Coombs test

   D. ANA

   E. Major cross-match

Bill is a 30-year-old man who presents with lower right quadrant abdominal pain, a 10-pound weight loss over the past month, fever, and nonbloody diarrhea. Barium enema contrast imaging indicates mucosal swelling of the wall of the ileum and ascending colon. A biopsy of the colon shows the presence of transmural granulomatous inflammation. Laboratory tests indicate mild anemia, leukocytosis, and decreased total serum protein and albumin, which suggest anorexia.

4. Which of the following therapies would be expected to be most beneficial in treating this condition?

   A. Plasmapheresis

   B. Anti-tumor necrosis factor (TNF)-α

   C. Recombinant C1 Inh

   D. Appendectomy

   E. Antifungal agents

A 72-year-old man complains of bilateral swelling and pain in the joints of his hands and feet. Several of his proximal phalangeal joints are noticeably deformed. A radiograph of the right hand shows a narrowing of the joint spaces in three digits.

5. Which of the following additional findings would support a diagnosis of rheumatoid arthritis?

   A. A decreased erythrocyte sedimentation rate

   B. Serum antibodies to double-stranded DNA

   C. Antibodies to IgG in the serum

   D. A positive response to antibiotics

   E. Autoantibody to the TSH receptor

ANSWERS

1. The correct answer is B. Acute episodes in lupus are accompanied by complement depletion by activation of the classical pathway. This leads to a decline in the serum levels of C1, C2, C3, and C4.

2. The correct answer is A. Over 95% of lupus patients have antinuclear antibodies. The other choices do not fit a diagnostic approach to autoimmunity, except choice E. Antibodies to myelin are typical of multiple sclerosis, but not SLE.

3. The correct answer is C. The most appropriate test for establishing an immune basis for an anemia is the Coombs test, which detects IgG antibodies on erythrocytes. This patient's fatigue is most likely related to her low erythrocyte mass.

4. The correct answer is B. This case fits the classic signs and symptoms of Crohn's disease and the imaging and laboratory data support this diagnosis. Chronic inflammation is maintained by the activation of a Th1 type of cytokine production, including IL-12,

interferon (IFN)-γ, and TNF-α. Anti-TNF-α has proven effective in treating Crohn's disease in many patients.

5. The correct answer is C. Although not diagnostic of this condition, the presence of rheumatoid factor certainly distinguishes rheumatoid arthritis from several other forms of arthritis. Lupus patients can develop arthritis, but the condition of not erosive in nature. *Increased* sedimentation rates are common in acute disease.

CHAPTER 17
TRANSPLANTATION

I. The **principles of transplantation** predict the survival of transplanted tissues.

    A. Tissue or organs transplanted within an individual are accepted.

        1. Such grafts are called **autografts**.

        2. Examples of autografts include skin transplants to treat local burns and cosmetic hair follicle transplantation to treat hair loss.

    B. Grafts exchanged between genetically identical individuals are accepted.

        1. These grafts are called **isografts**.

        2. The donor and recipient are **isogeneic** or **syngeneic** to one another.

    C. Grafts between genetically dissimilar individuals are rejected.

        1. The donor and recipient are **allogeneic** to one another.

        2. The grafts are referred to as **allografts**.

    D. Grafts exchanged between species are normally rejected.

        1. The donor and recipient are **xenogeneic**.

        2. The grafts are called **xenografts**.

    E. Foreign **histocompatibility antigens** initiate graft rejection.

        1. Major histocompatibility complex (MHC) alloantigens (ie, human HLA) are the strongest stimuli for inducing allograft rejection.

        2. Minor histocompatibility antigens and **tissue-specific antigens** can mediate graft rejection.

            a. Vascular endothelial cells express ABO antigens that can stimulate hyperacute rejection.

            b. Endothelium-specific antigens can trigger graft rejection.

        3. MHC alloantigens are recognized directly by large numbers of cross-reacting $CD4^+$ and $CD8^+$ T cells (Figure 17–1).

            a. Most T cell receptors (TCRs) cross-react with allogeneic forms of MHC.

            b. Up to 15% of all peripheral T cells can be activated by a single MHC alloantigen.

        4. Multiple MHC incompatibilities lead to more vigorous graft rejection than does a disparity at a single locus (Figure 17–2).

        5. Disparities at MHC class I + MHC class II loci induce greater responses than does either a class I or a class II difference alone.

        6. Prior immunization can increase the pace of allograft rejection.

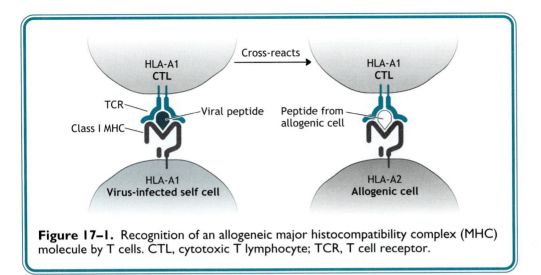

Figure 17–1. Recognition of an allogeneic major histocompatibility complex (MHC) molecule by T cells. CTL, cytotoxic T lymphocyte; TCR, T cell receptor.

    a. **"First set" rejection** occurs within days because the number of T cells activated by a foreign graft is large.

    b. Repeated exposure to the same MHC alloantigens (eg, through blood transfusions) can cause even more rapid rejection (**"second set" rejection**).

  F. The fate of allografts varies somewhat depending on the nature of the tissue or organ transplanted (Table 17–1).

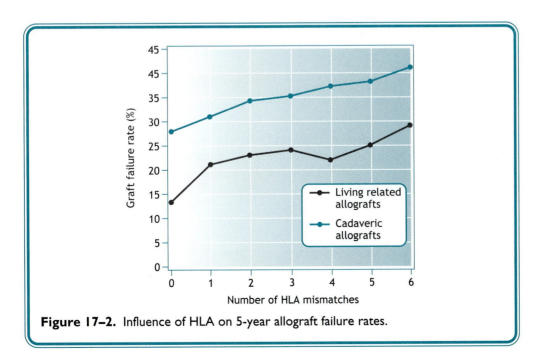

Figure 17–2. Influence of HLA on 5-year allograft failure rates.

Table 17–1. Special considerations related to particular forms of transplantation.

Organ or Tissue Transplanted	Considerations
Kidney	95% overall success rate after 1 year when living related kidneys are used; diabetes is the most frequent cause of end-stage renal failure
Heart	Reserved for imminently life-threatening cardiac disease; often combined with lung transplantation; relaxed criteria for donor selection due to organ shortage and effectiveness of cyclosporin
Lung	Low success rate compared to other solid organs
Blood	Transfusions are typically tolerated despite HLA disparity; preformed anti-HLA antibodies can cause transfusion reactions
Liver	Less requirement for HLA typing; evidence that tolerance to allogeneic transplants develops with time; contraindicated in certain malignancies, viral hepatitis, and human immunodeficiency virus (HIV) infection
Pancreas	Prevention of secondary effects of diabetes; whole organ, segmental, or isolated islet cell transplantation possible
Hematopoietic stem cells	Concern for graft-versus-host disease and infections; graft-versus-tumor effect beneficial
Cornea	Benefits from the privileged status of the anterior chamber

CORNEAL TRANSPLANTS

- *Approximately 40,000 corneal transplants are performed in the United States each year.*
- *The donors are not routinely matched with recipients for HLA, and recipients do not receive systemic immunosuppression following transplantation.*
- *The immunologically privileged status of the anterior chamber of the eye results in a low level of graft rejection (~10%).*
- *Immune privilege is maintained by a lack of lymphatic drainage and the expression of **Fas ligand** (Chapter 6) on corneal endothelial and epithelial cells.*
- *Invading activated T cells expressing Fas are killed by binding to ocular Fas ligand.*
- *When they occur, rejection episodes can be treated with topical corticosteroids.*

    II. Allograft rejection involves a diverse set of immune mediators (Figure 17–3).

        A. CD4⁺ Th1 cells activate various effector cells by secreting cytokines.

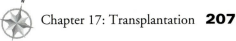

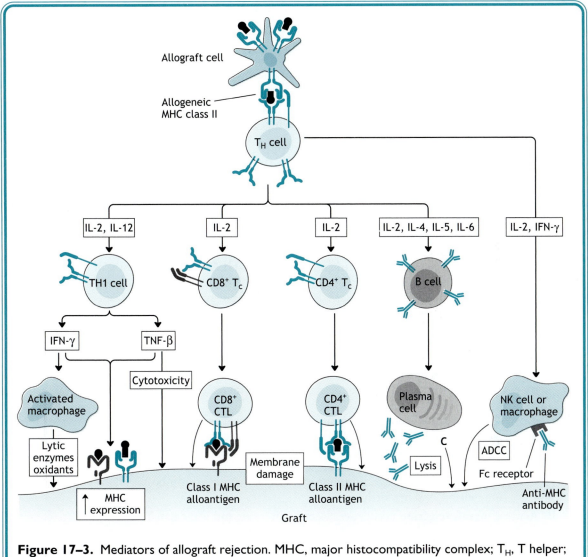

Figure 17–3. Mediators of allograft rejection. MHC, major histocompatibility complex; T$_H$, T helper; IL, interleukin; T$_C$, cytotoxic T cell; IFN, interferon; TNF, tumor necrosis factor; NK, natural killer; ADCC, antibody-dependent cell-mediated cytotoxicity.

1. Th1 cells recognize **allogeneic HLA-DP, DQ, and DR** molecules.
2. The Th1 cell subset produces interleukin (IL)-2, interferon (IFN)-γ, and tumor necrosis factor (TNF)-α, which activate cytotoxic T cells, natural killer (NK) cells, and macrophages.

B. **CD4+ Th2 cells** are activated by allogeneic MHC class II molecules.
   1. The Th2 cytokines IL-4 and IL-5 induce growth, class switching, and antibody production by B cells.

2. **Antibodies** specific for allogeneic donor MHC molecules can mediate **hyper-acute rejection** (see below).

3. Immunoglobulin (Ig) G alloantibodies can promote **antibody-dependent cellular cytotoxicity (ADCC)** by NK cells and macrophages.

C. **Cytokines** that mediate allograft rejection are also produced by NK cells (IFN-γ), CD8⁺ T cells (IFN-γ), and macrophages (TNF-α).

D. **CD8⁺ cytotoxic T cells** recognize allogeneic MHC class I molecules.

1. Killing is mediated by the perforin–granzyme, Fas–Fas ligand, and TNF receptor pathways (Chapter 10).

2. Rejection is due to apoptotic cell death in the transplanted tissues.

E. **Macrophages** kill donor cells with oxidants, hydrolytic enzymes, and TNF-α.

F. **NK cells** kill by recognizing the absence of self MHC class I molecules.

III. Three mechanisms of allograft rejection exist.

A. **Hyperacute allograft rejection** occurs within minutes to hours and is mediated by preformed antibodies in the recipient.

1. The principal target antigens include allogeneic HLA and ABO, both of which are expressed on the donor's vascular endothelial cells.

2. Anti-HLA antibodies are produced in response to pregnancy, blood transfusions, or prior transplants.

3. These IgM and IgG antibodies activate complement through the classical pathway.

a. C5a attracts neutrophils to the allograft.

b. iC3b promotes neutrophil attachment and activation.

c. C3a, C4a, and C5a activate mast cells, which increases the inflammatory response within the graft.

4. Activated neutrophils, monocytes, and NK cells damage the endothelium.

5. Activation and damage to the vascular endothelium cause important hemodynamic changes in the allograft.

a. Tissue factor is expressed by endothelial cells and initiates thrombosis.

b. Endothelial cell damage promotes platelet activation, thrombosis, infarction, edema, and hemorrhage.

B. **Acute allograft rejection** occurs over weeks to months and is mediated by CD4⁺ Th1 cells, CD8⁺ cytotoxic T cells, NK cells, and macrophages that infiltrate the graft.

C. **Chronic allograft rejection** occurs over months to years.

1. **Fibrosis, infarction, and ischemia** are common features.

2. Chronic rejection is difficult to control by immunosuppression.

IV. Graft rejection can be predicted or prevented by matching the donor and recipient histocompatibility antigens (Table 17–2).

A. **Tissue typing** determines the tissue antigens expressed by prospective donors and recipients and any preformed immunity to those antigens.

1. **ABO matching** is essential for preventing endothelial damage by isohemagglutinins.

2. Preformed antibodies to ABO are detected with the **major cross-match** (incubating donor cells in recipient serum).

Table 17–2. Prospective HLA typing for the transplantation of solid organ allografts.

	Mediator of Rejection		
	CD4⁺ Th Cells	**CD8⁺ Cytotoxic T Cells**	**Antibodies**
HLA antigens recognized	HLA-DP, DQ, DR	HLA-A, B, C	ABO; HLA-A, B, C, DP, DQ, DR
Important typing procedures	Type and match HLA-DP, DQ, DR Perform mixed lymphocyte reaction (MLR)	Type and match HLA-A, B, C	Major cross-match to detect anti-ABO and anti-HLA

TRANSPLANTATION ACROSS ABO INCOMPATIBILITIES

- *Conventional wisdom advises against transplanting organs when an ABO incompatibility exists between the donor and recipient.*
- *This restriction has limited the number of cardiac transplants, especially those involving infants with congenital heart defects.*
- *Recently, it was discovered that ABO incompatibility need not prevent the transplantation of HLA-matched hearts into very young children.*
- *The isohemagglutinins that mediate hyperacute rejection develop slowly over time in the neonate.*
- *The antigenic stimulus for inducing isohemagglutinins appears to be the cross-reacting polysaccharides of microbial flora.*
- *The delayed appearance of these natural antibodies reflects a gradual acquisition of commensal organisms during the initial months of postnatal life.*

    3. HLA typing is performed by molecular techniques [eg, polymerase chain reaction (PCR)].
        a. The best donor–recipient pair is selected based on similarities between their HLA genotypes.
        b. HLA typing and matching can minimize acute rejection.
        c. Extensive matching of HLA types is not as important in liver transplants as in kidney transplants (Table 17–1).
        d. The shortage of heart allografts and the effectiveness of cyclosporine in cardiac transplantation obviate the need for extensive HLA typing.
        e. HLA typing is important for identifying haplotype segregation within a family (Figure 7–7).
        f. Transplantation using organs from deceased donors may not afford an opportunity for detailed tissue typing.
        g. High-resolution typing of HLA-D region antigens is important in stem cell transplantation to avoid graft-versus-host disease (GVHD).
    4. Preformed anti-HLA antibodies are detected with a **major cross-match**.

a. Such antibodies can be formed against either class I or class II alloantigens.
    b. The major cross-match can prevent hyperacute rejection.
  5. The **mixed lymphocyte reaction (MLR)** detects T cell-mediated reactivity between donor and recipient (Figure 17–4).
    a. The assay measures the recognition of allogeneic MHC by coculturing the lymphocytes from two individuals.
    b. The MLR also predicts the potential for **GVHD** following stem cell transplantation.

TRANSPLANTATION WAITING LISTS

CLINICAL CORRELATION

- *Recent national data (www.ustransplant.org) indicate that over 80,000 patients in the United States are waiting for organ transplants, a number that has doubled in less than 10 years.*
- *Nearly 60,000 patients await kidney transplantation, while only 15,000 renal transplants are performed each year.*
- *Two-thirds of prospective kidney transplant recipients spend over a year on the waiting list.*
- *The median time until transplantation is over 3 years.*

  V. Xenotransplantation has the potential to address the shortage of available donor organs and tissues.
    A. The species providing a xenotransplant to a human patient is determined by organ physiology as well as social and ethical concerns.
      1. Kidneys from minipigs are suitable for transplantation into humans, based on anatomical and physiological considerations.
      2. Pigs are also suitable for genetic manipulation (see the Clinical Correlation on transgenic pigs in Chapter 8).
    B. Xenotransplantation carries the risk of transmitting **zoonotic infections**.
      1. Retroviruses similar to human immunodeficiency virus type 1 (HIV-1) are a particular concern.

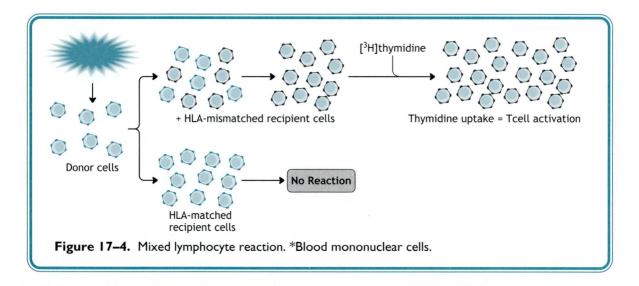

Figure 17–4. Mixed lymphocyte reaction. *Blood mononuclear cells.

2. Immunosuppressed transplant recipients are at increased risk for such infections.

C. The primary immunological barrier to xenotransplantation appears to be **hyperacute rejection**.
   1. Natural IgM antibodies against widely distributed ABO-like carbohydrate xenoantigens are present in nearly all species.
   2. These antibodies activate complement and initiate neutrophil-mediated damage to vascular endothelial cells.
   3. Because the membrane complement regulatory proteins [eg, decay-accelerating factor (DAF)] of the pig do not inhibit the human C3 convertases, uncontrolled complement-mediated damage also occurs.

D. T cells that recognize the MHC molecules of the xenogeneic species are also activated and mediate strong rejection responses.

VI. Hematopoietic stem cell (HSC) transplantation provides a therapy for hematopoietic disorders, immune deficiencies, and cancer (Table 17–3).

A. HSCs bear the **CD34** marker and can be purified from bone marrow cells.
   1. HSCs can also be purified from peripheral blood after mobilization in the donor by injection of **colony-stimulating factor-granulocyte (CSF-G)**.
   2. For the treatment of malignant conditions, autologous HSCs can be collected during remission and transplanted at a later time.

B. Several potential outcomes of stem cell transplantation must be balanced.
   1. **Rejection** of an HSC transplant can be minimized by tissue typing.
   2. **GVHD** represents a significant risk in HSC transplantation beginning at the first month posttransplantation.
      a. Acute GVHD presents as a sunburn-like rash, hepatosplenomegaly, jaundice, elevated billirubin, and diarrhea.
      b. GVHD occurs when the recipient expresses HLA antigens not present on the donor.

Table 17–3. Diseases treated by hematopoietic stem cell transplantation.

Defects in Hematopoiesis	Immune Deficiencies	Malignancies
Sickle cell disease	Severe combined immune deficiency	Acute myeloid leukemia
Thalassemia	Wiscott–Aldrich syndrome	Acute lymphoblastic leukemia
Aplastic anemia	Leukocyte adhesion defect	Chronic myelogenous leukemia
Pure red cell aplasia	Chediak–Higashi syndrome Hyper-IgM syndrome	Multiple myeloma

c. GVHD requires donor T cells capable of responding to allogeneic HLA of the recipient.

    d. GVHD is most evident when the recipient is immunosuppressed or genetically incapable of rejecting donor T cells.

    e. GVHD can be anticipated by tissue typing in the direction of donor anti-host.

  3. Despite the negative effects of GVHD, donor T cells can also have a beneficial **graft-versus-tumor effect** in malignant diseases.

  4. The use of preconditioning regimens (eg, chemotherapy prior to transplantation) and powerful immunosuppressive drugs increases the risks of **opportunistic infections**.

    a. Depending on the degree of myeloablation, early infections can be severe and can be caused by viruses, fungi, and bacteria.

    b. Common pathogens include cytomegalovirus, herpes simplex virus, *Candida albicans,* and *Aspergillus* species.

    c. Neutrophil functions are generally restored first.

    d. Prophylactic therapies include antimicrobial agents, laminar flow rooms, intravenous immunoglobulin (IVIG), and pediatric vaccines after lymphocyte reconstitution.

VII. Posttransplantation immunosuppressive therapy primarily targets lymphocyte activation, growth, and differentiation and inhibits inflammation (Table 17–4).

Table 17–4. Immunosuppressive drugs used in transplantation.[a]

Agents	Targets	Clinical Use
Irradiation	Many cells	Conditioning for stem cell transplantation
Methotrexate, azathioprine	Many cells	Organ transplantation, autoimmunity
Mycofenolate mofetil	Lymphocytes	Organ transplantation
Cyclosporine A (CsA), tacrolimus (FK506), sirolimus (rapamycin)	Lymphocytes	Organ transplantation
Corticosteroids	Many cells	Inflammatory diseases, organ transplantation
OKT3	T cells	Organ transplantation
ALG, ATG, daclizumab	Lymphocytes	Organ transplantation

[a]ALG, antilymphocytic globulin; ATG, antithymocyte globulin.

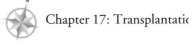

A. Cyclosporine and related drugs block calcineurin-dependent activation of nuclear factor of activated T cells (NFAT) in T cells and inhibit cytokine (eg, IL-2) production (Chapter 6).

B. Azathioprine and methotrexate are cytotoxic to lymphocytes.
  1. **Azathioprine** inhibits DNA synthesis.
  2. **Methotrexate** is a folate antagonist.
  3. The drugs are also used to treat autoimmune diseases (Chapter 16).

C. Antibodies against lymphocytes or their receptors block signaling and cause lymphocyte death.
  1. **OKT3** is an antibody to CD3 used in pancreas transplantation.
  2. **Antilymphocyte globulin** and **antithymocyte globulin** deplete T cells.
  3. **Daclizumab** is an antibody against the IL-2 receptor (CD25), which inhibits lymphocyte proliferation.

D. Corticosteroids inhibit inflammation (eg, neutrophil and macrophage activation) associated with graft destruction.

E. Mycophenolate mofetil inhibits purine metabolism and blocks lymphocyte proliferation.

F. All of these drugs are essentially nonspecific in the sense that they inhibit protective immune responses while suppressing graft rejection.

CLINICAL PROBLEMS

Mary is a 52-year-old woman with end-stage renal disease secondary to diabetes. She received an allogeneic renal transplant 2 months ago and has progressed to a maintenance dose of immunosuppressive therapy. However, within the last week she has been experiencing a progressive decline in renal function [decreased urine output, elevated blood urea nitrogen (BUN) and creatine] and currently has a temperature of 39°C. Her kidney is now tender, painful, and swollen. A renal biopsy shows a dense interstitial mononuclear infiltration.

1. Which of the following is most likely responsible for the change in her clinical course over the past week?

  A. An opportunistic viral infection

  B. Renal toxicity due to her immunosuppressive drugs

  C. Graft-versus-host disease

  D. Acute allograft rejection

  E. Diabetic nephropathy

Two months after having received an allogeneic stem cell transplant for the treatment of acute lymphoblastic leukemia, a patient presented with diarrhea and a blistering, erythematous appearance to the skin of his anterior neck and back. Serum chemistry revealed elevated liver enzymes and billirubin, and the liver and spleen appeared enlarged on physical examination.

2. Which of the following diseases or pathogenic mechanisms is most likely causing this clinical picture?

A. Rejection of the transplant

B. Autoantibody production against the patient's lymphocytes

C. Deposition of immune complexes in the skin and liver

D. A reaction to his immunosuppressive drugs

E. Graft-versus-host disease

As a treatment for end-stage renal disease, xenotransplantation involves unique clinical challenges not seen in allotransplantation.

3. Which of the following mechanisms is more common in the rejection of renal *xeno*grafts than renal allografts?

A. Production of IgE antibodies

B. Activation of HLA class I-restricted CD4$^+$ T cells

C. Binding of anti-HLA antibodies to donor tissues

D. Activation of complement by natural antibodies

E. Attraction of eosinophils into the graft

The HLA phenotypes of a family, including a patient who requires a kidney transplant, are listed below.

Family Member	HLA-A Alleles	HLA-B Alleles	HLA-DR Alleles
Mother	1,7	8,12	4,5
Father	5,7	28,32	4,6
Daughter #1	1,7	8,32	5,6
Daughter #2	1,7	8,28	4,4
Son #1	1,5	12,28	4,5
Son #2	1,7	12,32	5,6
Patient	**1,5**	**8,28**	**4,4**

4. All other considerations being equal, which of the family members is best suited as the transplant donor?

A. Daughter #1

B. Daughter #2

C. Mother

D. Son #1

E. Son #2

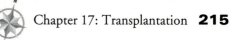

5. Which of the donors above would be most appropriate to donate *stem cells* to the patient if that were the indicated therapy?

   A. Daughter #1

   B. Daughter #2

   C. Mother

   D. Son #1

   E. Son #2

ANSWERS

1. The correct answer is D. This is a typical description of acute renal allograft rejection. The histopathology confirms rejection, but does not fit a virus infection or diabetic nephropathy (hyaline thickening of the glomerular capillaries).

2. The correct answer is E. GVHD is common in allogeneic stem cell transplantation and involves the liver, spleen, gastrointestinal tract, and skin.

3. The correct answer is D. Although allografts can also undergo hyperacute rejection initiated by isohemagglutinins, this rarely occurs due to the now routine use of the major cross-match. Hyperacute rejection is currently the major initial barrier to successful xenografting.

4. The correct answer is B. Daughter #2 has only a single disparity at one MHC class I locus. Particularly important in selecting a donor–recipient pair is avoiding disparities at both class I and class II loci.

5. The correct answer is B. The most important consideration in selecting a stem cell donor is avoiding GVHD, which is primarily induced by donor cells that recognize HLA-D region alloantigens of the recipient. The second consideration in selecting a donor for stem cell transplantation is the survival of the graft, which is dictated by the same rules that govern solid organ transplantation.

Appendix I. CD markers and their functions.[a]

CD Marker	Principal Functions
CD1	Presentation of glycolipids to NKT cells
CD3	Signaling chains of the TCR
CD4	Coreceptor for MHC class II-restricted T cells
CD8	Coreceptor for MHC class I-restricted T cells
CD11	α chain of the β_2 integrin family
CD14	Nonsignaling component of the LPS receptor
CD18	β chain of the β_2 integrin family
CD19	Signal transducer on B cells
CD20	Chain of the CR2 coreceptor
CD21	Chain of the CR2 coreceptor
CD25	α chain of the IL-2 receptor
CD28	Coreceptor on T cells that binds B7
CD34	Marker on hematopoietic stem cells
CD40	Coreceptor on B cells
CD45	Tyrosine phosphatase of T and B cells
CD55	Membrane decay accelerating factor
CD59	Membrane regulator of MAC assembly
CD80	B7-1 coreceptor on APCs
CD154	Ligand on T cells for CD40

[a]NKT, natural killer T; TCR, T cell receptor; MHC, major histocompatibility complex; LPS, lipopolysaccharide; IL, interleukin; MAC, membrane attack complex; APC, antigen-presenting cell.

Appendix II. Cytokines.[a]

Cytokine	Principal Functions
IL-1 α, β	Similar to TNF-α; fever, leukocyte adhesion, lymphocyte costimulation
IL-2	T, B, and NK cell proliferation
IL-3	Proliferation of progenitor cells; growth factor for mast cells
IL-4	Differentiation of Th2 cells and B cells; Ig class switching to IgE.
IL-5	Differentiation of B cells and eosinophils; Ig class switching to IgA
IL-6	Hematopoiesis, acute phase response
IL-7	Progenitor B and T cell growth
IL-8	Chemotaxis of neutrophils
IL-10	Inhibits the Th1 pathway
IL-12	Coactivator of the Th1 pathway; induces IFN-γ production
IL-13	Ig class switching to IgE
IL-15	NK cell growth
IL-18	Coactivator for IFN-γ production
TGF-β	Antiinflammatory; promotes wound healing; chemotaxis; Ig class switching to IgA
TNF-α	Proinflammatory; neutrophil and endothelial cell activation; proapoptotic
IFN-α,β	Inhibits viral replication; primes macrophages
IFN-γ	Macrophage activation; inhibition of Th2 pathway
CSF-M	Growth and differentiation of monocyte/macrophage lineage
CSF-G	Growth and differentiation of granulocytes
CSF-GM	Growth and differentiation of myeloid lineage cells

[a]IL, interleukin; TNF, tumor necrosis factor; NK, natural killer; Ig, immunoglobulin; IFN, interferon; TGF, transforming growth factor; CSF, colony-stimulating factor; M, macrophage; G, granulocyte. See also Table 12-3 for a list of important chemokines.

INDEX

Note: Page numbers followed by *f* or *t* indicate figures or tables, respectively.

Notes